Opiate Receptor Mechanisms

Neurochemical and Neurophysiological Processes in
Opiate Drug Action and Addiction

Based on a Work Session of the Neurosciences Research Program

by
Solomon H. Snyder
and
Steven Matthysse

with
Huda Akil, Ian Creese,
Peter A. Mansky, and Gavril W. Pasternak

Ava B. Nash and Joyce Taylor
NRP Writer-Editors

The MIT Press
Cambridge, Massachusetts, and London, England

The Neurosciences Research Program is sponsored by The Massachusetts Institute of Technology and is supported in part by National Aeronautics and Space Administration, National Institute of Mental Health Grant No. MH23132, National Institute of Neurological Diseases and Stroke Grant No. NS09937, National Science Foundation, Office of Naval Research, The Grant Foundation, Neurosciences Research Foundation, The Rogosin Foundation, and The Alfred P. Sloan Foundation.

This book is being published simultaneously as Volume 13, Number 1, February 1975, of the *Neurosciences Research Program Bulletin*.

This book was printed and bound in the United States of America.

ISBN 0-262-19132-6
Library of Congress catalog card number: 75-7828

CONTENTS

PARTICIPANTS

Huda Akil
Department of Psychiatry
Stanford University Medical Center
Stanford, California 94305

Floyd E. Bloom
Division of Special Mental Health
    Research Programs, IR, NIMH
William A. White Building
Saint Elizabeths Hospital
Washington, D.C. 20032

Ian Creese
Department of Pharmacology
    and Experimental Therapeutics
The Johns Hopkins University
    School of Medicine
725 North Wolfe Street
Baltimore, Maryland 21205

Pedro Cuatrecasas
Department of Pharmacology
    and Experimental Therapeutics
The Johns Hopkins University
    School of Medicine
725 North Wolfe Street
Baltimore, Maryland 21205

Vincent P. Dole
The Rockefeller University
York Avenue and 66th Street
New York, New York 10021

Mac V. Edds, Jr.
Neurosciences Research Program
165 Allandale Street
Jamaica Plain, Massachusetts 02130

Avram Goldstein
Addiction Research Foundation
701 Welch Road, Suite 325
Palo Alto, California 94304

Albert Herz
Max Planck Institute for Psychiatry
Clinical Institute
Kraepelinstrasse 2
8 Munich 40,
Federal Republic of Germany

John Hughes
Unit for Research on Addictive Drugs
Marischal College
Aberdeen AB9 1AS, Scotland

Leslie L. Iversen
Neurochemical Pharmacology Unit
Medical Research Council
Department of Pharmacology
Medical School
Hills Road
Cambridge CB2 2QD, England

Arthur E. Jacobson
National Institute of Arthritis and
    Metabolic Diseases
National Institutes of Health
Building 4, Room 137
Bethesda, Maryland 20014

Hans W. Kosterlitz
Unit for Research on Addictive Drugs
Marischal College
Aberdeen AB9 1AS, Scotland

Horace H. Loh
Department of Pharmacology
School of Medicine
University of California
San Francisco, California 94143

Arnold J. Mandell
Department of Psychiatry
University of California, San Diego
    School of Medicine
P.O. Box 109
La Jolla, California 92037

Peter A. Mansky
Psychiatric Research Laboratories
Massachusetts General Hospital
Boston, Massachusetts 02114

William R. Martin
Addiction Research Center
National Institute on Drug Abuse
P.O. Box 12390
Lexington, Kentucky 40511

Steven Matthysse
Psychiatric Research Laboratories
Massachusetts General Hospital
Boston, Massachusetts 02114

David J. Mayer
Department of Physiology
Medical College of Virginia
Box 608
Virginia Commonwealth University
Richmond, Virginia 23298

José M. Musacchio
Department of Pharmacology
New York University Medical Center
550 First Avenue
New York, New York 10016

Walle J.H. Nauta
Department of Psychology
Massachusetts Institute of
    Technology—Room E10-104
Cambridge, Massachusetts 02139

Gavril W. Pasternak
Department of Pharmacology
    and Experimental Therapeutics
The Johns Hopkins University
    School of Medicine
725 North Wolfe Street
Baltimore, Maryland 21205

Agu Pert
Psychology Group
Biomedical Laboratory
Edgewood Arsenal, Aberdeen
Proving Ground, Maryland 21010

Candace B. Pert
Department of Pharmacology
    and Experimental Therapeutics
The Johns Hopkins University
    School of Medicine
725 North Wolfe Street
Baltimore, Maryland 21205

Francis O. Schmitt
Neurosciences Research Program
165 Allandale Street
Jamaica Plain, Massachusetts 02130

Eric J. Simon
Department of Medicine
New York University Medical Center
550 First Avenue
New York, New York 10016

8

Solomon H. Snyder
Department of Pharmacology
   and Experimental Therapeutics
The Johns Hopkins University
   School of Medicine
725 North Wolfe Street
Baltimore, Maryland   21205

William H. Sweet
Massachusetts General Hospital
Boston, Massachusetts 02114

A.E. Takemori
Department of Pharmacology
University of Minnesota
   Medical School
105 Millard Hall
Minneapolis, Minnesota   55455

Lars Terenius
Department of Medical Pharmacology
Uppsala University
Box 573
S-751 23 Uppsala, Sweden

E. Leong Way
Department of Pharmacology
School of Medicine
University of California
San Francisco, California   94143

Frederic G. Worden
Neurosciences Research Program
165 Allandale Street
Jamaica Plain, Massachusetts   02130

Note: NRP Work Session reports are reviewed and revised by participants prior to publication.

I. INTRODUCTION

Opium and its derivatives have been used for centuries for a variety of medical and social reasons, but the mechanisms by which these drugs achieve their effects in the brain and on behavior have, until now, remained obscure. Several important new discoveries on the pharmacology, physiology, and biochemistry of opiate action prompted the need to air these findings in a cross-disciplinary setting and, accordingly, a group of some of the leaders in this field were brought together in an NRP Work Session. This review of the mechanisms of action of the opiate receptor reports the results of their discussions of ongoing investigations and attempts to place these disparate but converging findings within the broader context of neuroscience.

The criteria necessary for binding activity to be associated with a "receptor" were discussed intensively at the Work Session, and there was general agreement among the participants that the properties of opiate binding conform to the requirements of a "receptor."

The exquisite stereospecificity of the opiates and the availability of a graded series of agonists and antagonists have made the opiate receptor more tractable to research than most neurotransmitter receptors, and our understanding of this receptor may serve to increase our knowledge of other brain transmitters. The degree to which stereospecific opiate binding can be displaced by nonradioactive agonists and antagonists correlates remarkably well with their pharmacological potencies.

Since morphine is not a normal body constituent, what is the physiological function of the opiate receptor? A most remarkable development, first reported at this Work Session, is the finding that brain extracts from untreated animals contain a substance with morphine-like properties that binds to the opiate receptor and has naloxone-reversible, opiate-like effects on the mouse vas deferens and guinea pig ileum. The chemical structure of this proposed "endogenous ligand" is still largely unknown, although recent developments have opened up many possibilities for future research.

Another area of active exploration discussed at this meeting concerns the ability of sodium to distinguish neatly between opiate agonists and antagonists. The binding of agonists is decreased by sodium while the binding of antagonists is increased, enabling one to predict the agonist, antagonist, or mixed properties of a drug proposed for clinical use. The "sodium effect" is likely to be related to a conformational change in the receptor induced by the action of sodium on an allosteric site. It was proposed that a similar conformational change might be the basis of the addictive state, thus providing new clues for our understanding and treatment of the closely related and ٠ highly elusive phenomena of dependence and tolerance. The use of the simple, sensitive, and specific opiate receptor binding assay may well facilitate development of pure opiate antagonists for treating narcotic addiction and mixed agonist-antagonists with potential as nonaddicting analgesics.

Analgesia can be produced by implantation of opiates into selected brain regions, or by electrical stimulation under proper conditions. In general there is impressive convergence between the regions from which electrical and drug-induced analgesia is obtained and the brain areas, mostly confined to limbic structures, in which opiate-receptor binding is most concentrated. This regional distribution of the opiate receptor also closely parallels the motivational-affective pathways that mediate pain perception. It is also remarkable that electrically induced analgesia can be blocked by opiate antagonists and shows cross-tolerance to morphine. It was further conjectured that the endogenous ligand for the opiate receptor might be released by the circuits activated by electrically induced analgesia. This new knowledge may help to elucidate the neuroanatomical and physiological correlates of pain, thus providing new ways to relieve it.

Because the opiate receptor represents the initial site of drug action, the meeting focused selectively upon clarifying the interrelations between neural mechanisms thought to be closely linked to the receptor. Having restricted our goals in this way, we had to omit several important areas of opiate research, such as self-administration of drugs. Nonetheless, our enhanced understanding of opiate receptor mechanisms, the "first messenger," may enable researchers to discern second, third, and even fourth messengers and ultimately to elucidate the mediation of opiate analgesia, euphoria, tolerance, and physical dependence.

This introduction is intended to indicate some of the highlights of an unusually productive meeting. The reader new to this field may find the introductory sections on the chemistry and action of opiates, addiction, and pain, which provide background material, an especially helpful resource.

Chemistry of Opiates: A. Goldstein

Opium, the dried powder obtained from the milky exudate of the unripe seed capsules of the poppy plant, contains a number of active alkaloids. The compound responsible for most of opium's effect is morphine, which comprises about 10% (by weight) of the powder. Thebaine, an inactive alkaloid, which is an important precursor for commercial preparation of semisynthetic opiates, and codeine are also found in significant amounts. The long history and extensive use of morphine has led to the development of many semisynthetic and synthetic analgesics. One of the first of these, heroin, was obtained by acetylating the hydroxyl groups on morphine. Since then, many additional compounds have been synthesized from morphine and thebaine, and several completely new types of compounds have been designed. These new groups include the benzomorphans, such as pentazocine, the phenylpiperidines, such as meperidine, the diphenyl-amines, such as methadone, the morphinans, such as levorphanol, and the 6,14-endo-ethenyloripavines, such as etorphine.

Although these drugs differ widely in chemical structure, there are common features. The major features are a phenanthrene ring and a piperidine ring at right angles with a methyl substituent and a phenolic hydroxyl (Figure 1). Morphine is a T-shaped molecule with two broad hydrophobic surfaces at right angles, and a nitrogen that is protonated at physiological pH and carries a methyl group. The hydrophobic T-conformation is essential; the phenolic hydroxyl is capable of hydrogen bonding and the cationic nitrogen can form an ionic bond. If the phenolic hydroxyl is methylated, as in codeine, the molecule has no opiate activity.

Morphine can exist in several stereoisomeric forms of which only two are commonly prepared. Generally, pharmacological activity resides almost exclusively in the (−)-isomer of opiates; the (+)-isomers are usually devoid of analgesic activity. In the morphinan series, for example, levorphanol, the (−)-isomer, has all the analgesic activity whereas dextrorphan has none. This is illustrated in Figure 2 for the guinea pig ileum myenteric plexus/longitudinal muscle preparation, described in the section below, "Changes in Sensitivity to Neuro-transmitters in the Opiate-Tolerant Myenteric Plexus."

The search for more potent and less addictive analgesics has also resulted in the discovery of structurally similar drugs that reverse, or

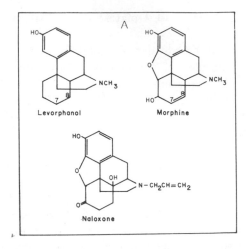

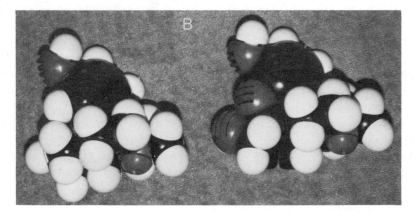

Figure 1. A. Structures of typical opiates. Levorphanol, at left, contains the main elements of the opiate structure as described in the text. Morphine, at right, contains additional, dispensable features such as an alcoholic hydroxyl group, an oxygen bridge, and an unsaturation at position 7-8. Naloxone is an antagonist; the N-allyl substituent confers this property. Naloxone is an analog of the agonist oxymorphone (see Figure 3). B. Stereochemical features of the opiate structure. Levorphanol at left, morphine at right. The molecules are positioned as in A, phenolic OH at upper left, nitrogen atom in planar hydrophobic surface at lower right. [Goldstein]

antagonize, the effects of morphine. These drugs, termed antagonists, usually differ from corresponding agonists by the substituent on the nitrogen. Some examples are nalorphine, naloxone, and levallorphan. In these three, a methyl group is replaced by an allyl group on the nitrogen. Cyclopropylmethyl nitrogen substitution (a group similar in

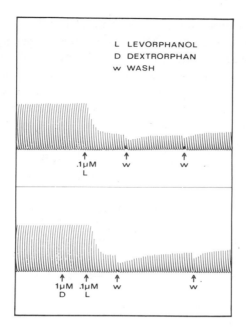

Figure 2. Stereospecificity of pharmacological action in the morphinan series. Record shows twitches of guinea pig ileum longitudinal muscle resulting from field stimulation of myenteric plexus (0.1 Hz). Upper record shows inhibition caused by 0.1 μM (final concn) levorphanol. Lower record shows inertness of dextrorphan, the (+)-isomer of levorphanol, at 10-fold higher concentration. Note that effect of levorphanol remains unchanged in presence of dextrorphan, i.e., the latter is not an antagonist. [Data of R. Schulz and A. Goldstein]

size to the allyl group) also produces antagonists. Paradoxically, larger substituents (e.g., ethylphenyl) again produce agonists.

Opiate Action
(This section prepared by P.A. Mansky)

There is an extensive literature, both literary and scientific, containing descriptions of the effects of opiates: subjectively perceived effects, observed behavioral changes, and physiological consequences (see, for example, De Quincey, 1822; Burroughs, 1962; Brown, 1965; Krueger et al., 1941; Reynolds and Randall, 1957; Haertzen, 1966).

Opiates act on both the peripheral and the central nervous system in man. Description of the phenomenology of their actions is important for suggesting hypotheses about mechanisms underlying each effect.

Most complex are the gross behavioral changes observed after opiate administration in man. Although opiates are generally considered behavioral depressants, one often sees an increase of activity in certain species after opiate administration. This increase in activity has also been observed in non-opiate-dependent postaddicts who describe a "drive" or increased motivation after receiving opiates (Fraser et al., 1963). Observers have also noted increased verbal activity in the same subjects at doses of morphine varying from 10 to 30 mg/70 kg. The sleep seen after opiate administration is sometimes described as "twilight sleep" from which one can easily be awakened (Kay et al., 1969).

In low to moderate doses, opiates promote feelings of relaxation and sedation; at higher doses, opiates produce stupor and coma but leave intact some reactions to environmental stimuli. Thus a subject, who by many measures appears comatose and unresponsive to pain and to both the hypercapnic and anoxic respiratory drives, will breathe if the command to breathe is given.

Although opiates can produce behavioral depression and coma, they do not elicit general central nervous system depression. Sedative hypnotics also produce coma and behavioral depression while dramatically increasing the seizure threshold, whereas opiates actually induce seizures in man at high doses and, in some species, at surprisingly low doses.

More specific but still difficult to explain mechanistically are the euphoriant and analgesic effects of opiates. Although some investigators claim to be able to measure morphine-like euphoria in a dose-related fashion (Haertzen, 1966), Goldstein objected to the use of the term "euphoria" for an effect more properly described as an extraordinary change in mood producing oblivion to external stimuli.

Kolb (1925) described the ability of opiates to produce euphoria, using terms analogous to behavioral positive- and negative-reinforcement paradigms. Thus negative euphoria occurs when a person feels that a drug restores him to normality from a state of chronic dysphoria. Positive euphoria occurs if a drug enables people, already feeling normal, to feel better or high. Although these concepts are vague, they do allow for speculation concerning the mechanism of drug action.

Even more sophisticated is the morphine-benzedrine group scale derived from the 500 items in the Addiction Research Center Inventory (ARCI), which gives a dose-related response grading to morphine and contains items that a priori suggest a sense of well-being or improved function. This scale is affected in a dose-related manner by both morphine and amphetamine.

Although opiates consistently produce euphoria in some people, others find the effects of opiates to be distinctly unpleasant. An interesting study was carried out by Lasagna, von Felsinger, and Beecher (1955) in Boston and Isbell at the Addiction Research Center (ARC). Both groups of subjects received amphetamine and morphine in a double-blind crossover experimental design. The Boston subjects were naive to the effects of opiates and amphetamines, whereas the subjects at the ARC were experienced drug users. The ARC subjects stated that they enjoyed both amphetamine and opiates although they tended to rate the opiates as more pleasant. The Boston subjects enjoyed amphetamine but disliked opiates.

Some of the dysphoria associated with morphine may derive from a decreased ability to think clearly. In the study by Lasagna and his colleagues, the personality profile of the Boston subjects revealed strong intellectual and academic drive. They might have experienced the morphine-induced mental clouding as dysphoric. By contrast, the ARC former addicts might not regard a state of diminished alertness as unpleasant. The vegetative effects of morphine, such as nausea and vomiting, urinary retention, and smooth muscle spasm in the intestines, ureter, and cystic duct may account for the dysphoria of many patients who dislike opiates even though the drugs relieve their pain.

The relative ability of various opiates to produce euphoria in postaddicts correlates well with their relative analgesic activity measured in clinical settings (Beaver et al., 1969; Forrest, 1970, 1972; Houde et al., 1970, 1972; Jasinski and Mansky, 1970, 1972). Opiate analgesia is generally thought to result from both altered perception of painful stimuli and an alteration in the affective or "feeling" reactions to pain.

Besides inducing analgesia, opiates elicit a wide range of effects in numerous bodily functions. Depending on the situation, these effects may have important clinical utility or may just become troublesome side effects.

Pupillary constriction is a prominent effect of opiates in man. As Bloom pointed out during the meeting, miosis appears to be almost species specific for man. Nauta noted that respiratory depression with pupillary constriction is virtually diagnostic of opiate overdose. Although local application of morphine to the eye will produce pupillary constriction (Nomof et al., 1968), pupillary constriction in man is predominantly mediated by the brain.

Morphine also has prominent effects on the respiratory system. Bloom pointed out that morphine appears to block the hypercapnic drive for respiration in the medullary centers. Only in much higher doses does morphine depress the anoxic drive.

Morphine and other opiates are antitussive in subanalgesic doses, although this is not a stereospecific effect and is most likely related to brainstem actions (Chakravarty et al., 1956). Nonetheless, the antitussive actions of opiates are of great therapeutic importance. Dextromethorphan, the analgesically inactive (+)-isomer of a potent opiate, is the most widely used "cough medicine" in the United States.

Opiates in general decrease glandular secretions and contract smooth muscles. Both of these effects are prominent in producing constipation or treating diarrhea, depending on the patient's disposition. Morphine appears to prevent coordinated regular intestinal peristalsis and also to contract smooth muscle. These effects, coupled with decreased gastrointestinal secretions and decreased central appreciation of rectal fullness, lead to constipation (Bogoch et al., 1954; Paton, 1957; Daniel et al., 1959; Gyang and Kosterlitz, 1966; Hopton and Torrance, 1967).

Similar smooth muscle effects upon the urinary bladder and sphincters along with central stimulation of antidiuretic hormone (ADH) may lead to decreased urinary output and may produce acute urinary retention. Occasionally the detrusor muscles are stimulated, resulting in both increased urgency and the inability to void. Contraction of the sphincter of the gall bladder increases pressure in the bile ducts and can result in pain resembling biliary colic.

The nausea and vomiting seen with opiate administration in man appear related to the firing of neurons in the chemoreceptor trigger zone (CTZ), which Bloom pointed out is a vaguely defined group of medullary neurons that triggers the emetic center. Occasionally nausea and vomiting are diminished by large doses of morphine used in surgical anesthesia. Conceivably these large doses of morphine depress the CTZ and prevent it from activating the emetic center.

The incidence of nausea and vomiting produced by opiates is greater in ambulatory than in bedridden patients. This phenomenon may be related to vestibular stimulation of nausea and vomiting mechanisms when patients move about. Thus, unlike the nausea and vomiting produced by sedative-hypnotic drugs, opiate-induced nausea and vomiting are relieved by bed rest. Therefore, both exogenous vestibular stimulation and CTZ stimulation appear to be important in producing nausea and vomiting.

Interestingly, opiate-naive subjects have a higher incidence of nausea and vomiting after opiate administration than nonaddicted, experienced opiate users, which, together with a greater decrease in rectal temperature, are the only physiological differences seen between the groups (Fraser and Isbell, 1952).

Of clinical value in recognizing opiate intoxication is the itching of the skin and nose-rubbing it induces. This little-understood effect may result from histamine release from mast cells. Histamine release by opiates has also been proposed as the mechanism for dramatic drug-induced decreases in blood pressure. Although a pronounced fall in blood pressure is not frequent, orthostatic hypotension occurs often after opiate administration (Drew et al., 1946).

Goldstein indicated that opiates cause hypothermia, which can be produced (or antagonized) by microinjection into the anterior hypothalamus. Opiates also block release of thyroid-stimulating hormone (TSH). It is interesting that this effect can be blocked by lesions that by themselves do not alter TSH release, suggesting that the opiate effect is on a modulatory pathway (Lomax and George, 1966).

Addiction
(This section prepared by P.A. Mansky)

The word "addiction" is used frequently to refer to properties of opiates that are related to promoting their continued self-administration in animals and in man. As such, "addiction" appears to be synonymous with "drug dependence" as presently defined by the World Health Organization (WHO) Expert Committee on Drug Dependence.*

To understand terms used to connote drug dependence, one can examine historically the definition of terms used by the WHO committee and also look at changes in the pattern and description of drug-use phenomena during the same time.

*Formerly, WHO Expert Committee on Addiction-Producing Drugs.

In its seventh report, the committee defined addiction and habituation as follows:

> *Drug addiction* is a state of periodic or chronic intoxication produced by the repeated consumption of a drug (natural or synthetic). Its characteristics include: (1) an overpowering desire or need (compulsion) to continue taking the drug and to obtain it by any means; (2) a tendency to increase the dose; (3) a psychic (psychological) and generally a physical dependence on the effects of the drug; (4) detrimental effect on the individual and on society.
>
> *Drug habituation (habit)* is a condition resulting from the repeated consumption of a drug. Its characteristics include: (1) a desire (but not a compulsion) to continue taking the drug for the sense of improved well-being which it engenders; (2) little or no tendency to increase the dose; (3) some degree of psychic dependence on the effect of the drug, but absence of physical dependence and hence of an abstinence syndrome; (4) detrimental effects, if any, primarily, on the individual. [WHO Expert Committee on Addiction-Producing Drugs, 1957, p. 9]

Addiction and habituation seem to connote two different poles of drug use, one being pernicious and difficult to alter, the other being less harmful to the individual and society and more easily treated or changed.

According to these definitions, physical dependence is not absolutely required for a diagnosis of "addiction," but it is usually present. During the late 1950's and early 1960's, several drug-use patterns were emerging that failed to conform to the above definitions. Amphetamine can produce marked psychological dependence with no physical dependence. Conversely, a class of drugs known as narcotic antagonists (nalorphine and cyclazocine) were found to produce physical dependence but no drug craving (Martin et al., 1966).

In non-opiate-dependent subjects, nalorphine produces a unique constellation of subjective effects. Low doses (1 to 5 mg) elicit mild euphoria and analgesia, while higher doses (3 to 10 mg) produce a combination of sedative-hypnotic and psychotomimetic effects that are considered by most subjects to be dysphoric. The effects of high doses resemble being "overtired"; that is, feeling tired but unable to sleep because of the excitant effects of the drugs. Subjects appear drunk or ataxic and drowsy, but cannot sleep enough to feel rested.

These subjective effects decrease upon repeated drug administration. If the dose is increased slowly, large amounts of the antagonists can be administered with complete tolerance to their subjective and physiological effects. When the drugs are withdrawn, an abstinence syndrome occurs resembling that seen with opiates. The subjects, however, experience no opiate- or other drug-seeking behavior during the abstinence period (Martin et al., 1966). Thus, for opiate antagonists, physical dependence can occur without drug craving. By contrast, drugs such as amphetamines promote compulsive drug use in certain individuals without producing physical dependence.

In 1969, the WHO Expert Committee on Drug Dependence substituted the term "drug dependence," the sine qua non of which was psychological dependence, for the terms "addiction" and "habituation"; they adopted the following definitions:

> *Drug dependence:* A state, psychic and sometimes also physical, resulting from the interaction between a living organism and a drug, characterized by behavioural and other responses that always include a compulsion to take the drug on a continuous or periodic basis in order to experience its psychic effects, and sometimes to avoid the discomfort of its absence. Tolerance may or may not be present. A person may be dependent on more than one drug.
>
> *Physical dependence capacity:* The ability of a drug to act as a substitute for another upon which an organism has been made physically dependent, i.e., to suppress abstinence phenomena that would otherwise develop after abrupt withdrawal of the original dependence-producing drug. [p. 6]

Isbell and Chruściel (1970) offered the following additional definitions:

> *Psychic dependence:* A compulsion that requires periodic or continuous administration of a drug to produce pleasure or avoid discomfort. This compulsion is the most powerful factor in chronic intoxication with psychotropic drugs, and with certain types of drugs may be the only factor involved in the perpetuation of abuse even in the case of most intense craving. Psychic dependence, therefore, is the universal characteristic of drug dependence. Operationally, it is recognized by the fact that the dependent continues to take the drug in spite of conscious admission that it is causing harm to his health and to his social and familial adjustment, and that he takes great risks to obtain and maintain his supply of the drug.

20

Physical dependence: A pathological state brought about by repeated administration of a drug and that leads to the appearance of a characteristic and specific group of symptoms, termed an abstinence syndrome, when the administration of the drug is discontinued or—in the case of certain drugs—significantly reduced. In order to prevent the appearance of an abstinence syndrome the continuous taking of the drug is required. Physical dependence is a powerful factor in reinforcing psychic dependence upon continuing drug use or in relapse to drug use after withdrawal.

Tolerance: The state in which repetition of the same dose of a drug has progressively less effect, or in which the dose needs to be increased to obtain the same degree of pharmacological effect as was caused by the original dose.

Cross-tolerance: The state in which tolerance to one drug has the effect of causing tolerance to another drug of the same or a different chemical type. [Isbell and Chruściel, 1970, p. 5]

The use of the term "drug dependence" as defined above with a modifying phrase linking it to a particular type of drug was supported by the WHO Scientific Group on Evaluation of Dependence-Producing Drugs (1964) and has also been supported by the Committee on Drug Addiction and Narcotics of the National Academy of Sciences—National Research Council (see Eddy et al., 1965).

Thus drug dependence, according to these definitions, is a behavioral response resulting from both the properties of certain drugs and the psychological makeup of particular individuals. Physical dependence is important in that it can reinforce the state of psychological dependence.

Pain
(This section prepared by H. Akil)

Opiates are used by the clinician primarily to relieve severe pain resulting from a wide variety of causes. Although chronic use will eventually lead to tolerance and dependence in a patient, opiates remain the most powerful pharmacological tool available for the production of analgesia.

The analgesic property of opiates has been the focus of numerous animal studies aimed at elucidating the site and mechanism of action of these drugs in the central nervous system. This endeavor is complicated by the fact that pain is a subjective phenomenon, and its physiological substrates remain obscure. At one level, it can be seen as a basic and primitive response signaling tissue damage to the organism; as such, it is essential for survival. Its pathways within the central nervous system are wired in what appears to be a redundant fashion.

Although pain is thought of as a sensation resulting from any tissue-damaging stimulus to the organism, it is obvious that it has strong emotional components not usually present in such sensations as audition or touch. In fact, many workers define a "painful" stimulus operationally as one that the animal escapes or avoids either reflexively or through learned responses. Pain is often contrasted to pleasure as both an emotion and a drive state.

Any pain response is likely to involve sensory input that codes the presence of the noxious stimulus, limbic components mediating emotional properties of the response, and motor system events leading to the withdrawal reflex or escape response. There are major disagreements about the details of each of the above three components, particularly the sensory coding and the limbic involvement. Whereas some scientists believe that pain, like all other sensations, requires specific peripheral receptors, others insist that it is merely a function of the *pattern* of sensory input. Thus, Perl (1972) and Iggo (1959) find that terminals of some of the small nonmyelinated C fibers are receptors in the skin that transmit thermal or mechanical information in a specific fashion; that is, only when the stimulus is intense enough to produce pain. On the other hand, Melzack and Wall (1965) are strong proponents of a pattern theory in which C fibers facilitate the processing of pain input, while the larger, faster fibers tend to inhibit pain. Their "gate control theory" emphasizes the interactions between different types of sensory input and explains certain observations of the inhibition of pain by nonpainful input, such as rubbing the skin or applying a cold stimulus.

The pathways into the brain are not well understood beyond the level of the thalamus. Their terminations in the cerebral cortex are unknown, and their interactions with limbic structures remain obscure. Even the mechanisms involved in the simplest withdrawal reflex at the spinal cord level appear exceedingly complex.

A further source of confusion is the fact that pain responses are highly variable from subject to subject and are a function of the general emotional state of the individual. Beecher (1946) reported that wounded soldiers in the field who expected to return home because of their wounds appeared to feel no pain, whereas they responded normally to other noxious stimuli under other conditions. The fact that pain can be inhibited by changes in perception, by hypnosis, or when other survival matters appear more urgent has suggested the presence of a pain-inhibitory mechanism in the brain that interacts with input and modifies the perception and response. Casey and Melzack (1967) postulated that such a system would descend into the spinal cord and alter the pattern of input at the "gate."

However, the most difficult problem facing investigators is to provide a model for what is termed "chronic" pain. Phenomenologically, noxious stimuli that are fast and short lived, like a pinprick, are termed "acute" pain. Others are slow, possibly less intense, but longer lasting, like the aftermath of a burn. In many clinical cases, pain can last for months or years and is termed "chronic" pain. There is some evidence that acute and chronic pain are mediated by somewhat different mechanisms in the brain. The majority of animal studies are performed with acutely noxious stimuli, but opiates are primarily used to alleviate the deeper, slower type of pain.

The numerous elements involved in the processing of pain render its study in the laboratory difficult. Pain is never directly measured; rather we measure a response to a noxious input. Changes in that response are taken to indicate changes in the pain sensation. Thus, the choice of the pain measure is crucial. Spinal reflexes are more reliable and easier to measure but may not fully reflect changes in emotional and perceptual components. On the other hand, complex pain responses are easily modified by factors such as learning, memory, or emotions, and changes may not necessarily reflect alteration in the pain sensation itself.

Nonetheless, across a wide range of responses, types of pain, situations, and species, opiates appear to alter responsivity to pain. Given the view that both sensory and emotional elements are involved in pain processing, where are opiates likely to act? Conceivably, they could *interrupt* the flow of sensory information from the periphery into the brain. Obversely, they could exert their analgesic action by *activating* the pain-inhibitory system that modulates the transmission of noxious input. Finally, they may alter the interpretation of *emotional* components of pain by reducing the accompanying anxiety or producing an effect similar to the "It hurts but I don't care" response seen in frontal lobotomized patients. There is no a priori reason to favor any one of these three hypotheses. It is in fact highly likely that morphine alters all aspects of the pain experience. However, some recent data appear to favor active inhibitory mechanisms as a major mode of action of pain blockade with opiates (Satoh and Takagi, 1971a,b).

Until recently, the investigation of opiate analgesia stood at the intersection of two extremely complex areas: the mechanisms of action of the drugs and the physiological mechanisms of pain. Finding a starting point appeared impossible. Recent breakthroughs identifying biochemically the pharmacologically relevant opiate receptor may provide a handle for understanding pain mechanisms in general, from both the anatomical and the neurochemical viewpoints.

II. BIOCHEMICAL IDENTIFICATION OF RECEPTORS

Criteria for Receptors: V.P. Dole, P. Cuatrecasas, and A. Goldstein

As a prelude to the theme of "the opiate receptor," Dole emphasized that objections could be raised to each of the three words, "the," "opiate," and "receptor." Although it is clear that there are binding sites with intriguing specificity, there is not yet proof that the binding site—opiate complex is biologically active. Stereospecificity may not be a sufficient condition for biological activity. Stereospecific binding might occur by chance, a not unlikely possibility considering, for example, the number of antibodies that are ready in advance to react with molecules never before encountered. The high affinity of the binding site is also not proof of functional activity; the binding constant should be appropriate to the biological concentration in the neighborhood of the receptor. Because opiates have multiple physiological actions (see section above, "Opiate Action"), even the word "the" should be used cautiously.

Cuatrecasas critically discussed the concept of "receptor." A receptor has two major functions. The first is recognition of the ligand, and the second is mediation of a biological response. In studies of ligand-receptor binding, there are several important criteria that must be satisfied, especially in the case of naturally occurring substances. The first is specificity, both pharmacological and steric. Second is saturability, implying that the number of receptors is limited. A third criterion is target-cell specificity. Binding should be observed on the same cells that exhibit a biological response. The affinity for the ligand must be appropriate with regard to the normally occurring or pharmacological concentration of the substance or hormone. Receptor binding should be reversible, consistent with the reversibility of the biological response.

An ancillary criterion supporting the biological relevance of the receptor is perturbation, such that changing the chemical structure of the receptor changes the biological response. Isolation of the receptor and reconstitution of the biological response is the ideal, seldom-achieved state.

Each of these criteria alone is not sufficient. Stereospecificity might be deceptive. D-Tryptophan binds stereospecifically to serum albumin. Saturability is relative, and all sorts of nonspecific binding may be saturable. Examples include the saturable, very high affinity binding of insulin to glass culture tubes, and the stereospecific binding of ^{3}H-naloxone to glass fiber filters (see below, Table 1).

All these criteria must be examined with reference to a particular biological response. With some hormones and drugs there may be multiple biological responses, many of which are difficult to measure in isolated systems. This poses a particularly perplexing problem with opiates.

Goldstein expanded on the criterion of stereospecific binding. Stereospecificity might be obtained in a system in which only one isomer can bind to the receptor. Alternatively, both isomers might bind to the receptor, but only one might have an effect. In the latter case, the inactive isomer should be a drug antagonist. Since the inactive dextro-isomers of opiates are not opiate antagonists, it is clear that the stereospecificity of opiate action occurs at the binding of the drugs to the receptor site. Goldstein and his collaborators (1971) suggested that opiate receptors might be identified by measuring stereospecific binding to brain tissue of radioactive opiates and first demonstrated such binding to membranes in mouse brain homogenates, using levorphanol and its isomer dextrorphan. Emphasizing specific binding, in this case stereospecific binding, is important because opiates, like many psychotropic drugs, are very lipophilic and will bind nonspecifically to biological membranes. Stereospecific binding is a necessary, but not sufficient, condition for identifying pharmacologically relevant opiate binding.

Why should there be a specific receptor site for opiate narcotic drugs? This question could be posed for many drugs. Some, like general anesthetics, might act pharmacologically by altering membrane functioning in a diffuse, nonspecific fashion, as is suggested by the lack of rigorous structural requirements for their actions. By contrast, despite some leeway, opiates all conform to a particular chemical structure (Figure 3). Moreover, some opiates exert their effects in extremely small doses. Etorphine is 5,000 to 10,000 times more potent than morphine in relieving pain in animals and in man. Another reason for suspecting that a specific opiate receptor exists is the dramatic stereospecificity of opiate action. For most opiates, only the levorotatory (−)-isomer exerts analgesic action. The existence of opiate antagonists also argues for a specific opiate receptor. Antagonists such as naloxone (Narcan) occupy opiate receptor sites, producing no effect

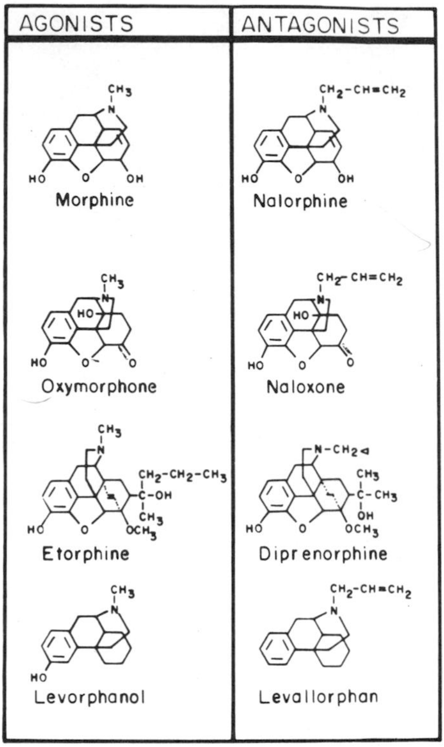

Figure 3. Structural comparison of 4 opiate agonists and antagonists. [Pert, 1974]

themselves but preventing the action of subsequently administered opiates. Opiate antagonists may have great importance, both in treating heroin addicts and in developing relatively nonaddicting analgesics. For all these reasons, it has generally been assumed that opiates exert their pharmacological effects by interacting with selective receptor sites in the brain.

Membrane Receptor: S.H. Snyder and C.B. Pert

Using labeled opiates or antagonists of high specific activity and washing samples after incubation to remove loosely bound and unbound radioactivity, Pert and Snyder (1973a), Simon and his co-workers (1973), and Terenius (1973a,b) independently identified binding to brain tissue that was highly stereospecific. These observations have since been confirmed by a number of other laboratories, including Hitzemann and Loh (1973), Wong and Horng (1973), Lee and his colleagues (1973), and Klee and Streaty (1974). However, as already mentioned, stereospecificity of binding, while necessary, is not a sufficient condition for identifying the opiate receptor. Because most body constituents are symmetrically disposed, it would be perfectly possible for naturally occurring substances, apparently unrelated to the opiate receptor, to bind opiates stereospecifically. In fact, Pasternak and Snyder* demonstrated stereospecific binding of ^{3}H-naloxone to glass fiber filters (Table 1). Initially they thought that they had solubilized the receptor from rat brain membrane fractions, but when controls without tissue were employed, it became evident that the results were attributable solely to stereospecific opiate binding to the filters.

TABLE 1

Glass Fiber Filter Binding of ^{3}H-Naloxone [Pasternak and Snyder]

	^{3}H-Naloxone bound (counts/min)			
	No drug	Levorphanol	Dextrorphan	Stereospecific
Solubilized receptor	815 ± 40	690 ± 15	862 ± 23	172 ± 27
Solubilized receptor (from trypsinized tissue	834 ± 24	603 ± 32	893 ± 53	290 ± 62
Buffer alone	1101 ± 51	579 ± 12	872 ± 30	293 ± 32

To obtain further evidence relating ^{3}H-naloxone binding to the pharmacologically relevant opiate receptor, Pert and Snyder evaluated a wide range of drugs (Table 2). In general there is a close parallel between the pharmacological potency of various opiates in producing or antagonizing analgesia and their affinity for the naloxone binding sites. Potent opiates such as morphine and levorphanol have affinities in the nanomolar range, whereas weak opiates such as meperidine (Demerol) and propoxyphene (Darvon) have much less affinity for the receptor.

There are some apparent discrepancies. Etorphine, which is thousands of times more potent than morphine in vivo, has only about 20 times the affinity of morphine for the receptor. However, etorphine is able to enter the brain from the general circulation 300 times as efficiently as morphine (Herz and Teschemacher, 1971). These two

*G.W. Pasternak and S.H. Snyder, unpublished observations.

28

TABLE 2

Relative Potencies of Drugs in Reducing Stereospecific
[3]H-Naloxone Binding to Rat Brain Homogenate [Pert and Snyder, 1973b]

Drug	ED_{50} (nM)	No effect at 0.1 mM
(−)-Etorphine	0.3	Phenobarbital
(−)-Etonitazene	0.5	Norepinephrine
Levallorphan	1	Atropine
Levorphanol	2	Pilocarpine
(−)-Nalorphine	3	Arecholine
(−)-Morphine	7	Colchicine
(−)-Cyclazocine	10	γ-Aminobutyric acid
(−)-Naloxone	10	Bicuculline
(−)-Hydromorphone	20	Serotonin
(−)-Methadone	30	Carbamylcholine
(±)-Pentazocine	50	Neostigmine
(+)-Methadone	300	Hemicholinium
Meperidine	1,000	Histamine
(±)-Propoxyphene	1,000	Glycine
(+)-3-Hydroxy-N-allyl-morphinan	7,000	Glutamic acid
Dextrorphan	8,000	Δ9-Tetrahydrocannabinol
(−)-Codeine	20,000	Acetylsalicylic acid
(−)-Oxycodone	30,000	Caffeine

Values represent means from 3 log-probit determinations, each using 5 concentrations of drug. ED_{50} = concentration of drug required to inhibit stereospecific ^{3}H-naloxone binding by 50%.

properties of etorphine explain a 6,000-fold difference in pharmacological potency in vivo. Similarly, codeine, which in vivo is about one-sixth as potent as morphine, is extremely weak in binding to the opiate receptor, with less than 1/2,000 the affinity of morphine. But abundant evidence indicates that codeine as such does not act directly in relieving pain but only after metabolic conversion by O-demethylation to morphine (Way and Adler, 1962). Thus codeine, though an effective analgesic when injected intraperitoneally to animals, has no action when administered directly into the brain (Adler, 1963).

To further ensure the specificity of the opiate receptor, Pert and Snyder examined the effects of a wide range of nonopiate drugs on receptor binding. None of them has any affinity for the opiate receptor even in concentrations as high as 0.1 mM (Table 2).

A particularly critical test of the pharmacological relevance of opiate receptor binding demands a homologous series of opiates of widely varying analgesic potencies. The ketobemidones, evaluated by Snyder's and May's laboratories (Wilson et al., 1975b), provide a series

TABLE 3

Binding and Analgesic Data [Wilson et al., 1975b]

Compound	Hot-plate analgesic (mM) ED_{50}	Inhibition of ^{3}H-naloxone binding (1 nM) ED_{50}		Ratio $\frac{+NaCl}{-NaCl}$
		No sodium	100 mM Sodium	
Methyl	2.1 (1.4-2.8)	7-10	70	7-10
Ethyl	67.2 (52.0-87.0)	400	1500-2000	3.8-5
Propyl	16.0 (13.2-19.1)	200	800-1000	4-5
Butyl	4.6 (3.8-5.9)	50	600-700	12-14
Pentyl	0.78 (0.62-1.0)	8	30	3.8
Hexyl	7.5 (5.5-10.3)	20	40	2
Heptyl	9.0 (7.0-11.6)	20	40-50	2-2.5
Octyl	26.5 (20.2-34.9)	200	200	1
Nonyl	inactive	700	700	1
Decyl	inactive	500	600-700	1.2-1.5

For hot-plate analgesic 95% confidence limits are shown in parentheses; ED_{50} = nM concentration of drug required to inhibit stereospecific ^{3}H-naloxone binding by 50%. Binding was performed using mouse brain homogenates. Eight mice were used at each dose and a minimum of 5 doses for each compound was used.

in which small alterations in side-chain length elicit dramatic variations in analgesic potencies and corresponding alterations in opiate receptor affinity (Table 3).

In determining whether the stereospecific binding of opiates in membrane preparations is pharmacologically relevant to opiate action, the ideal situation would be to compare directly affinities in the binding situation to potency in an in vitro pharmacological/physiological system. The guinea pig ileum provides such a possibility. Narcotic agonists stereospecifically inhibit the electrically induced contraction of the longitudinal muscle/myenteric plexus of the guinea pig ileum; narcotic antagonists reverse this inhibition. Kosterlitz's group has demonstrated that the potency of numerous opiates in this system correlates extremely well with their relative potency for analgesic action in man (Kosterlitz et al., 1973b; Kosterlitz and Waterfield, 1975). Creese and Snyder (1975) have been able to assay opiate receptor binding in both homogenates of this system (as previously reported by Terenius, 1972, 1973c; Pert and Snyder, 1973a) and mince preparations in which the tissue was intact in physiological buffers identical to those used to assess pharmacological activity. Opiates show

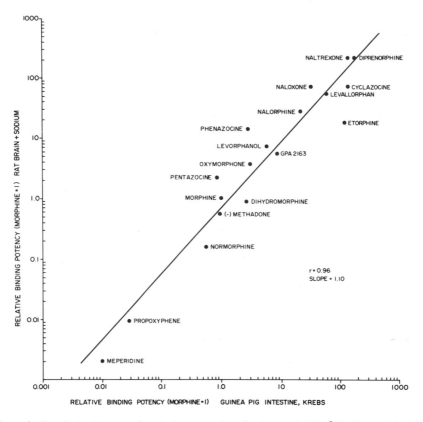

Figure 4. Correlation between the relative potencies of opiates to inhibit ^{3}H-naloxone binding in guinea pig intestine and rat brain homogenates. The relative potencies of opiates were calculated from ED_{50} determinations for each drug to inhibit stereospecific ^{3}H-naloxone binding in either homogenates of the guinea pig intestine longitudinal muscle/myenteric plexus preparation (assayed in Krebs-Tris, 37°C, pH 7.4) or homogenates of rat brain (assayed in 0.05 M Tris + 100 mM NaCl, 25°C, pH 7.7). The ED_{50} for morphine was taken as the standard in each system and given the value of 1. [Creese and Snyder, 1975]

stereospecific binding with affinities closely approximating those found in the rat brain when assayed with 100 mM Na$^+$ (Figure 4). The dissociation constant (K_D) for naloxone is the same whether the homogenate or tissue mince preparation is used. There is remarkable agreement between the kinetic parameters determined by receptor binding assay and measurements of opiate effects on electrically induced intestinal muscle contraction (Figure 5) (correlation co-efficient = 0.98). This demonstrates that the affinity of opiates for binding to the receptor is sufficient to explain their relative potency in causing a physiological response; that is, the binding receptor is the

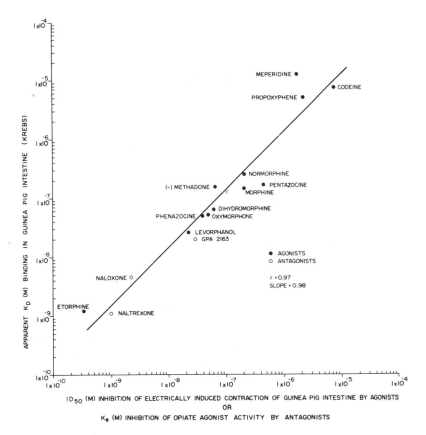

Figure 5. Correlation between receptor binding and pharmacological activities of opiates in the guinea pig intestine. The K_D, as determined by the inhibition of stereospecific ^{3}H-naloxone binding in homogenates of the guinea pig intestine longitudinal muscle/myenteric plexus preparation, for a series of opiate agonists and antagonists is plotted against the ID_{50} concentration, for agonists, required to inhibit the electrically induced contractions of the guinea pig intestine longitudinal muscle/myenteric plexus preparation by 50%, or the K_e, for antagonists, required to inhibit agonist activity in the same preparation. [Creese and Snyder, 1975]

physiologically active receptor. Furthermore, because of the close approximation in these kinetic parameters, receptor occupation is sufficient to explain the observed physiological response, and concepts such as efficacy, intrinsic activity, and spare receptors may not be necessary to account for opiate action.

In initial studies with relatively low specific activity naloxone, its affinity constant was about 20-60 nM (Pert and Snyder, 1973b). More recent studies by Pasternak and Snyder (1975) with higher specific activity naloxone reveal in addition a binding site with 50 to

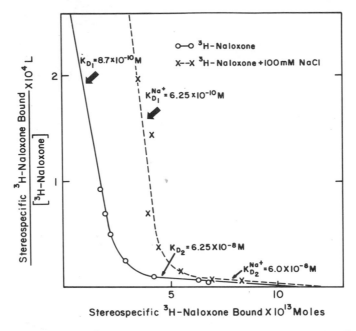

Figure 6. Scatchard plots of ^{3}H-naloxone binding in the presence and absence of NaCl: Two ml aliquots of brain homogenate (70 vol) were assayed in triplicate at 25°C for 30 min with varying concentrations of ^{3}H-naloxone in the presence and absence of 100 mM NaCl and either (−)- or (+)-3-hydroxy-N-allyl-morphinan at 0.1 μM. [Pasternak and Snyder, 1975]

100 times the affinity of that initially reported. Scatchard plots of ^{3}H-naloxone binding, both in the presence and absence of sodium, describe curves that can be resolved into two linear components with K_D values of 0.6-0.9 nM and 60 nM for high- and low-affinity binding respectively (Figure 6). Including 100 mM sodium in the incubation medium doubles the number of apparent high-affinity binding sites, does not alter the number of low-affinity sites, and has no significant effect on the dissociation constants. The increase in ^{3}H-naloxone binding elicited by sodium will be described in greater detail in the section below, "Differential Interactions of Agonists and Antagonists with the Opiate Receptor."

Biphasic Scatchard plots are also obtained for ^{3}H-dihydro-morphine binding (Figure 7). In the absence of sodium, high-affinity binding for ^{3}H-dihydromorphine has a dissociation constant of about 0.5 nM, and low-affinity binding exhibits a dissociation constant of about 8 nM. Sodium (50 mM) virtually abolishes the ·high-affinity binding of ^{3}H-dihydromorphine and reduces the low-affinity binding

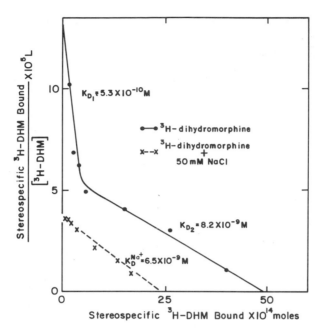

Figure 7. Scatchard plots of ^{3}H-dihydromorphine (^{3}H-DHM) binding in the presence and absence of NaCl: Two ml aliquots of brain homogenate (150 vol) were assayed in duplicate at 25°C for 30 min with varying concentrations of ^{3}H-dihydromorphine in the presence and absence of 50 mM NaCl and either (−)- or (+)-3-hydroxy-N-allyl-morphinan at 0.1 μM. All values for binding are stereospecific. [Pasternak and Snyder, 1975]

by about 50% without significantly altering its dissociation constant. In additional experiments, this decrease in ^{3}H-dihydromorphine low-affinity sites varies from 10% to 40%. Thus the effects of sodium on the binding of opiate agonists and antagonists are exerted predominantly upon high-affinity binding components.

In earlier studies, when higher concentrations of ^{3}H-naloxone (about 8 nM) were bound to brain homogenates, Pert and Snyder (1973b) found a half-life for dissociation of 5 min at 5°C, determined by displacing ^{3}H-naloxone with 10 μM nonradioactive naloxone. When dissociation is measured after incubation with 1 nM ^{3}H-naloxone and examined at 0°C, the half-life for dissociation is about 50 min (Figure 8) (Pasternak and Snyder, 1975). When 1 nM nonradioactive naloxone is added to the diluted incubation medium, the rate of dissociation accelerates and evinces a half-life of about 35 min. Dissociation is even more rapid with a half-life of about 28 min in the presence of 1 μM nonradioactive naloxone (Figure 8). Since the

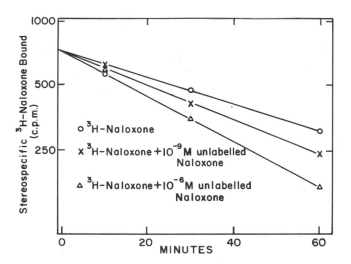

Figure 8. Dissociation of ^{3}H-naloxone in the presence and absence of unlabeled naloxone. Brain homogenate (50 vol) was prepared and bound with 1 nM ^{3}H-naloxone at 25°C for 30 min with either (−)- or (+)-3-hydroxy-N-allyl-morphinan at 0.1 μM. The homogenate was centrifuged (49,000 × g × 20 min at 0°C) and the pellet resuspended (time zero) in 10 times the original volume with the appropriate amount of unlabeled naloxone. Aliquots were incubated for the specified time at 0°C and then filtered and counted. All values for binding are stereospecific. The same dissociation rates with and without added naloxone were obtained in 5 separate experiments. [Pasternak and Snyder, 1975]

accelerated dissociation elicited by low concentrations of nonradioactive naloxone is probably not due to rebinding (Pasternak and Snyder, 1975), it probably reflects a negative cooperative interaction of naloxone with opiate receptor sites.

The two components in Scatchard plots for naloxone and dihydromorphine binding represent discrete high- and low-affinity binding functions. Because sodium has a fairly selective effect on the binding of naloxone and dihydromorphine to the high-affinity site, the high- and low-affinity binding functions appear to differ in some ways. Because binding of opiate agonists and antagonists to the receptor in the presence of sodium predicts their pharmacological activity, it is likely that the high-affinity binding component is more pharmacologically relevant than the low-affinity one.

The two binding components might be explained, at least in part, by negative cooperative interactions with the receptor indicated by the opiate-induced acceleration of receptor dissociation, as suggested for insulin by De Meyts and his co-workers (1973). However, the ability of protein reagents to destroy selectively high-affinity binding sites strongly suggests distinct sites (Pasternak et al., 1975).

Regional Distribution of the Opiate Receptor:
S.H. Snyder and C.B. Pert

A number of brain regions have been implicated in the perception of pain. Major ones are the rapidly conducting primary sensory pathways and the multisynaptic, slowly conducting, medially located paleospinothalamic and spinoreticular pathways. The latter involve areas of the brain such as the periaqueductal gray, the medial nuclei of the thalamus, the hypothalamus, and other regions comprising the limbic system. To determine the density of opiate receptors throughout the brain, Snyder's group measured receptor binding in numerous regions of monkey and human brain (Table 4) (Kuhar et al., 1973). Receptor binding varies by a greater than 30-fold range throughout the monkey brain. The amygdala shows the greatest amount, with its anterior portion displaying almost twice as much as the posterior. Binding in the periaqueductal area of the midbrain is about the same as in the posterior amygdala. The hypothalamus and medial thalamus, the next highest areas, display only about 40% as much binding as the anterior amygdala. No regional variations are detected within the hypothalamus, whereas the medial thalamus possesses about three times as much binding as the lateral thalamus. In the head of the caudate, receptor binding is about 80% of that in the hypothalamus and medial thalamus. Levels of binding in the putamen are similar to those of the hippocampus, the superior colliculi, interpeduncular nucleus area, frontal pole and superior temporal gyrus of the cerebral cortex. Within the cerebral cortex there are marked regional variations. Thus, binding in the precentral gyrus, postcentral gyrus, and occipital pole is less than a quarter of that in the frontal cortex. Receptor binding is very low or not detectable in various white matter areas. Receptor binding is also very low in the cerebellum, the lower brainstem, and the spinal cord. Receptor binding is quite similar in the human and monkey brains (Hiller et al., 1973; Kuhar et al., 1973).

What might this pattern of regional distribution indicate? Most brain biochemicals are distributed rather uniformly throughout the brain. The striking heterogeneity of opiate receptor distribution is reminiscent of the large regional differences for concentrations of neurotransmitters. There are similarities of opiate receptor distribution to the distribution of several neurotransmitters, such as acetylcholine, γ-aminobutyric acid (GABA), serotonin, and the catecholamines. However, there are differences as well. Thus, while acetylcholine and

TABLE 4 Opiate Receptor Binding in Regions of Monkey Brain [Adapted from Kuhar et al., 1973]

Region	Stereospecific dihydromorphine binding (fmol/mg protein)		Region	Stereospecific dihydromorphine binding (fmol/mg protein)	
Cerebral hemispheres			Extrapyramidal areas		
Frontal pole	11.9 ± 1.4	(4)	Caudate nucleus (head)	19.4 ± 2.3	(4)
Superior temporal gyrus	10.8 ± 2.5	(3)	Caudate nucleus (body)	9.0 ± 1.2	(3)
Middle temporal gyrus	7.1	(1)	Caudate nucleus (tail)	8.9 ± 3.0	(3)
Inferior temporal gyrus	6.0	(1)	Putamen	11.7 ± 1.9	(6)
Precentral gyrus	3.4	(2)	Globus pallidus	7.7	(2)
Postcentral gyrus	2.8	(2)	Internal capsule	5.4	(2)
Occipital pole	2.3 ± 0.5	(4)			
White matter areas			Midbrain		
Corpus callosum	<2	(2)	Superior colliculi	10.6 ± 2.0	(3)
Corona radiata	<2	(2)	Inferior colliculi	6.7 ± 0.7	(3)
Anterior commissure	5.4	(2)	Interpeduncular nucleus area	13.7 ± 1.5	(4)
Fornix	<2	(2)	Raphe area	8.2	(2)
Optic chiasm	<2	(2)	Periaqueductal gray	31.1 ± 4.6	(4)
Limbic cortex			Cerebellum-lower brainstem		
			Pons (ventral)	1.4	(2)
Anterior amygdala	65.1 ± 21	(4)	Cerebellar cortex	<2	(2)
Posterior amygdala	34.1 ± 4.2	(4)	Dentate nucleus	1.9	(2)
Hippocampus	12.5 ± 2.2	(4)	Floor of fourth ventricle	6.3 ± 1.3	(3)
Hypothalamus			Pyramidal tract	3.0	(2)
Medial hypothalamus	24.2 ± 3.2	(4)	Lower medulla	5.8	(2)
Anterior hypothalamus	24.3 ± 3.7	(3)			
Posterior hypothalamus	24.7 ± 1.4	(3)	Spinal cord (thoracic)		
Hypothalamus	23.2	(1)	Dorsal column (white)	3.1	(2)
Mammillary bodies	5.0	(1)	Lateral cord (white)	3.3	(1)
Thalamus			Gray matter	8.8	(2)
Medial thalamus	24.6 ± 1.6	(3)			
Lateral thalamus	7.8	(2)			

Values represent the mean ± SEM followed in parentheses by the number of determinations. Each determination was calculated from triplicate incubations with 1 nM ^{3}H-dihydromorphine in the presence of 100 nM levorphanol or dextrorphan. Five rhesus monkeys (*Macaca mulatta*) were decapitated 2 h after anesthesia with 30 to 45 mg/kg of sodium pentobarbital injected intraperitoneally. The brain was removed within 5 min and dissected rapidly on ice.

opiate receptor binding are both high in the caudate nucleus, the putamen is quite rich in acetylcholine but contains only moderate opiate receptor binding. The periaqueductal area of the midbrain, which possesses the second highest opiate receptor values, has only moderate acetylcholine-synthesizing capacity. Whereas the hypothalamus is rich in both GABA and opiate receptor, the globus pallidus, which contains one of the highest GABA concentrations in the brain, is relatively low in opiate receptor binding. Similarly, the occipital cerebral cortex contains more GABA than the frontal cortex, while their relationship is reversed for opiate receptor binding (Fahn and Côte, 1968). Like the opiate receptor, tyrosine hydroxylase, the enzyme that synthesizes the catecholamines norepinephrine and dopamine, is high in the caudate nucleus. The hypothalamus and periaqueductal gray are also rich in tyrosine hydroxylase and opiate receptor binding. However, while the medial thalamus contains much more opiate receptor binding than the lateral thalamus, the reverse situation holds for tyrosine hydroxylase. Serotonin is enriched in the caudate, hypothalamus, and amygdala, just as is the opiate receptor. However, the midbrain raphe area, which contains the cell bodies of serotonin neurons in the brain and is one of the richest areas in serotonin content, is quite low in opiate receptor binding.

Another way of determining whether the opiate receptor is associated with a specific neurotransmitter-containing neuron, is to make selective lesions of particular neurotransmitter-specific neuronal pathways. Lesions that selectively destroy norepinephrine-, serotonin-, acetylcholine-, or dopamine-containing pathways have no effect on opiate receptor binding in the areas of the brain in which these pathways possess the greatest density of nerve terminals (Kuhar et al., 1973).* This indicates that the opiate receptor is not contained on or within the nerve terminals of the specific pathways examined. It does not, however, rule out the possibility that the opiate receptor is localized to postsynaptic receptor sites for these pathways.

These regions and others rich in opiate receptor binding are all portions of the limbic system. Even the head of the caudate, which in the present dissection includes the nucleus accumbens, would qualify as a component of the limbic system. Similarly, the frontal and superior temporal cerebral cortices are more closely associated with the limbic system than other areas of the cerebral cortex and contain four to five times more receptor binding than other parts of the cerebral cortex.

*Also, I. Creese, personal communication.

38

Opiate receptor binding is, however, not uniformly high throughout the limbic system, since the mammillary bodies and hippocampus respectively possess low- and moderate-binding activity. Opiate receptor distribution corresponds fairly closely to the paleospinothalamic and spinoreticular pathways that may mediate motivational-affective components of pain.

Subcellular Localization

With a simple receptor assay, one can also ask questions about the localization of the receptor within cells of the brain. By differential and sucrose gradient centrifugation, it is possible to separate subcellular constituents of the brain. In homogenates of rat brain, opiate receptor binding is most enriched in the synaptosomal fraction, which contains primarily pinched-off nerve-ending particles (Figure 9) (Pert et al., 1974b). It is possible to evaluate discretely the interior components of nerve endings. One subjects the synaptosomal fraction to hypotonic shock and centrifuges the lysed material through a sucrose density gradient, providing fractions enriched in synaptic vesicles, synaptic membranes, mitochondria, and unruptured synaptosomes. Opiate receptor binding is recovered primarily in the synaptic membrane fraction with little, if any, receptor binding in the synaptic vesicle fraction. Interestingly, the opiate receptor binding of the nuclear fraction does not appear to be contained within nuclei themselves, because, when these are purified, they contain no opiate receptor binding. Instead, the opiate receptor occurs in membrane fractions that sediment with the nuclear pellet.

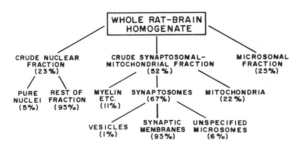

Figure 9. Subcellular distribution of stereospecific opiate receptor binding. The proportion of opiate binding in each fraction is indicated as percent of the binding of the parent fraction. [Snyder]

Narcotic Receptors in Guinea Pig Ileum and Rat Brain:
L. Terenius

The results described by Terenius are in general agreement with those obtained in the parallel studies by Snyder and by Simon and their co-workers, although Terenius used a somewhat different experimental approach. He used enriched membrane preparations from organ homogenates, balanced salt solutions, and, specifically, very highly labeled ^{3}H-dihydromorphine. Separation of bound and free dihydromorphine was done, without changing the equilibrium, by centrifugation; in later studies a rapid microassay was used (Terenius, 1974b).

Terenius (1973b) found the specific opiate binding to be localized in a fraction of rat brain enriched in synaptic plasma membranes. The pharmacological significance of the binding was studied by comparing analgesically effective doses (ED_{50}) with the doses needed to displace binding (IC_{50}). The correlations are good, especially for enantiomeric analogs of methadone as shown in Table 5.

The great importance of affinity for the biological activity is not unexpected because two optical antipodes should have nearly equal access to the receptor. On the other hand, for opiates with widely

TABLE 5

Receptor Affinities in Rat Brain Synaptic Membranes
Compared with Reported Analgesic Activities of
Methadone Analogs [Terenius, 1974b]

Substance	Affinity		Analgesic activity*	
	IC_{50}(M)†	Relative activity	ED_{50}(mg/kg)	Relative activity
6R-Methadone	4×10^{-9}	100	0.8‡	100
6S-Methadone	1×10^{-7}	4	25.2‡	3
Normethadone	2×10^{-8}	20		35§
3R,6R-Methadol	1×10^{-5}	0.04	63.7‡	1
3S,6S-Methadol	7×10^{-8}	6	3.5‡	23
3R,6S-Methadol	1×10^{-6}	0.4	24.7‡	3
3S,6R-Methadol	3×10^{-8}	13	7.6‡	11
Dextromoramide	5×10^{-9}	80	0.87‖	92
Levomoramide	4×10^{-6}	0.1	85‖	1

*Eddy hot-plate data for subcutaneous injection in mice.
†IC_{50} = concentration giving 50% inhibition of binding.
‡Eddy et al., 1952.
§Calculated; reported value relative to racemic methadone (Hardy and Howell, 1965).
‖de Jongh and van Proosdij-Hartzema (1957).

different physicochemical properties, differences in pharmacokinetics would be of considerable importance for the biological activity (Terenius, 1974a).

Other compounds tested with regard to ^{3}H-dihydromorphine binding include dopamine, norepinephrine, serotonin, histamine, acetylcholine, and Substance P, which fail to displace the labeled opiate at 10^{-5} M concentration. However, p-chloromercuribenzoate (1 mM), N-ethylmaleimide (1 mM), proteolytic enzymes, Triton X-100 (0.001%), and deoxycholate (0.001%), all decrease stereospecific ^{3}H-dihydromorphine binding (Terenius, 1973c).

Stereospecific binding can also be observed in brain slices (Figure 10). In the slices, binding that is depressed by the dextro-enantiomers (dextrorphan and dextro-methadone) is probably non-specific. The relevant binding is the difference between the levo-enantiomers and the respective dextro-enantiomers.

Receptor studies on the myenteric plexus/longitudinal muscle preparation of the guinea pig ileum were initiated because this preparation should provide a well-defined source of opiate receptors

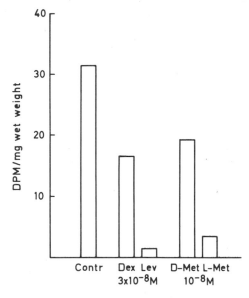

Figure 10. Stereospecific uptake of dihydromorphine to brain slices. Brain slices, nominally 0.3 mm thick from cerebral cortex, were incubated in physiological buffer of pH 7.4 (Terenius, 1974b) with 1 nM ^{3}H-dihydromorphine alone (Contr) or with addition of dextrorphan (Dex), levorphanol (Lev), dextro-methadone (D-Met) or levo-methadone (L-Met). Incubations were at 25°C for 40 min. Differences between the effects of respective enantiomers were significant at $p < 0.001$ (5 slices/group). [Terenius]

(Kosterlitz, this meeting). As previously reported, a high-affinity site for opiates is present in the crude mitochondrial preparation of this tissue (Terenius, 1972, 1973c). There is a good correlation between the affinity of drugs for this receptor and their biological potency (Table 6). Results in guinea pig ileum and rat brain also agree with Snyder's studies (Table 7). In Terenius's experiments, most drugs have about twice the affinity in the ileum as in the brain.

The binding assay was used in the search for an endogenous ligand for the opiate receptor. Organic solvent extracts of brain were

TABLE 6

Relation Between Receptor Affinity and Biological Activity
on Guinea Pig Ileum [Terenius]

Agent	IC_{50} (nM)	ID_{50} (nM)	K_e (nM)	$\dfrac{ID_{50}}{IC_{50}}$	$\dfrac{K_e}{IC_{50}}$
Morphine	3	68.2	87.5	23	29
Codeine	500	10,300	8,840	21	18
Levorphanol	0.6	9.18	7.04	15	12
Dextromoramide	1	6.68	4.33	6.7	4.3
Naloxone	0.4	>68,000	1.22	–	3.2

IC_{50} calculated as in Table 7; ID_{50} = morphine-like activity; K_e = naloxone-like activity; data for ID_{50} and K_e obtained from Kosterlitz and Watt (1968).

TABLE 7

Relative Affinity of Various Narcotic Analgesics for Guinea Pig
Ileum and Rat Brain Receptors [Terenius]

Agent	Ileum IC_{50} (nM)	Brain IC_{50} (nM)	Brain/ileum IC_{50}
Morphine	3	5	1.7
Codeine	500	700	1.4
l-Methadone	2	4	2.0
d-Methadone	50	100	2.0
Levorphanol	0.6	3	5.0
Dextrorphan	50	100	2.0
Dextromoramide	1	5	5.0

The assays were carried out according to Terenius (1974b). Incubates were the crude mitochondrial fraction from the myenteric plexus/longitudinal muscle of the guinea pig ileum or a synaptic plasma membrane fraction of rat brain. Nonspecific binding was subtracted from all values. Concentrations for 50% inhibition (IC_{50}) of the specific binding of ^{3}H-dihydromorphine (0.8 nM) were calculated from 4 to 5 mean values of quadruplicate determinations at 3 log-unit concentration differences. Assays on the 2 receptors were run simultaneously.

always negative regardless of the pH of the water phase, thus excluding any morphine-like agents. However, water extracts were positive. Terenius described the properties of an apparent endogenous ligand that has been isolated in his laboratory (Terenius and Wahlström, 1974) from acid water extracts of rat or calf brain homogenates. It has a molecular weight below 1,200 and it is water soluble and heat stable. The ligand is present in the cerebrum but is not found in the cerebellum. It reversibly inhibits the binding of ^{3}H-dihydromorphine in a dose-dependent manner. Most assays have been run with the synaptic plasma membrane receptor from brain rather than with the crude mitochondrial receptor preparation from the guinea pig ileum because the ligand is evidently degraded by the latter (Figure 11).

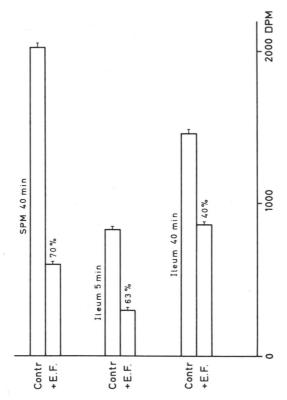

Figure 11. Effects of an endogenous factor (E.F.) isolated from rat brain (Terenius and Wahlström, 1974) on stereospecific binding of ^{3}H-dihydromorphine to opiate receptor in brain (synaptic plasma membrane (SPM) fraction) or ileum. The concentration of ^{3}H-dihydromorphine was 1 nM. Incubation with SPM-receptor for 40 min, with ileum receptor as indicated. The amount of E.F. used in the experiment is equivalent to 5 rat brains. The inhibition in all groups was significant at p < 0.001. [Terenius]

Opiate Receptor Binding with ^{3}H-Etorphine:
E.J. Simon

Simon, who uses ^{3}H-etorphine and ^{3}H-naltrexone for his binding studies on the membrane fractions of rat brain, presented data on the sensitivity of binding to various protein reagents and enzymes. The results were in very good agreement with those of Pasternak and Snyder (1974) and Terenius (this meeting). Simon found that prostaglandins E_1 and E_2, in concentrations up to 10^{-7} M, have no effect on opiate binding. The reason these compounds were tested was the report by Ehrenpreis and his colleagues (1973) that E prostaglandins antagonize inhibition by opiates of electrically induced contraction of isolated guinea pig ileum. These authors have suggested that the opiate receptor may be identical to the prostaglandin receptor. More recently, Collier and Roy (1974) have reported that opiates specifically inhibit the stimulation by prostaglandins of adenyl cyclase in rat brain homogenate.

Stereospecific binding of etorphine was studied by Simon and his collaborators (Hiller et al., 1973) in 40 anatomical regions of human brain obtained at autopsy. There were large variations in binding levels, ranging from 0.4 pmol bound/mg protein in the olfactory trigone and the amygdala to virtually no binding in the cerebellum, cerebral white matter, and endocrine glands. Most regions with high binding are those associated with the limbic system. A summary of these results is represented in Table 8. They are in good agreement with similar data obtained by Kuhar and his co-workers (1973) in monkey brain.

Since publication of these results, etorphine binding has been studied in 8 additional human brains. A number of new areas were surveyed. The highest binding group now also includes the insula, uncus, fusiform gyrus, and locus coeruleus. Moderate binding was observed in the cingulate gyrus and the paracentral lobule. The anterior portion of the cingulate gyrus was consistently higher than the posterior portion. Similarly, binding was found to be higher in the anterior hypothalamus than in the posterior portion. In preliminary experiments, opiate binding was measured in brain homogenates of heroin addicts and no difference from those of nonaddicts was reported. However, Pasternak pointed out that it is difficult to wash out opiates from brain tissue, and the morphine present in the brains of addicts, especially those dead from opiate overdose, would inhibit

44

TABLE 8

Grouping of Human Brain Regions According to Etorphine
Binding Capacity [Hiller et al., 1973]

High binding (0.44-0.23 pmol/mg protein)

Olfactory trigone*	Centromedian nucleus of thalamus*
Amygdala*	Preoptic area and supra optic nucleus*
Septal nuclei*	Cingulate gyrus*
Supra orbital gyrus of frontal lobe*	Dorsomedian nucleus of thalamus*
Parahippocampal gyrus*	Frontal lobe cortex*
Periventricular gray matter*	Pulvinar of thalamus
Temporal lobe*	

Moderate binding (0.21-0.15 pmol/mg protein)

Caudate nucleus	Olfactory bulb
Parietal lobe cortex	Periaqueductal gray
Hypothalamus*	Putamen
Ventral anterior nucleus of thalamus	Ventral posterolateral nucleus of thalamus

Low binding (0.12-0.07 pmol/mg protein)

Occipital lobe cortex	Cerebellar cortex
Corpora quadrigemina	Pretectum
Hippocampus*	Substantia nigra
Globus pallidus	Area postrema

Very low binding (0.05-0 pmol/mg protein)

Mammillary bodies	Olives
Medullary sensory nuclei	Dentate nucleus of cerebellum
Cerebral white matter	Tegmentum of mid pons
Posterolateral nucleus of thalamus	Pineal gland
Red nucleus	Pituitary gland

*Indicates components of the limbic system or regions associated with the limbic system.

binding in normal assays. Simon agreed that the failure to wash the brains extensively precludes definitive conclusions.

The marked inhibition of etorphine binding by increasing salt concentration (Simon et al., 1973) and the complete absence of such inhibition for naloxone binding (Pert and Snyder, 1973a) led Simon and his co-workers (1973) to postulate that this may represent a general difference in the manner in which agonists and antagonists bind to receptors. This was shown to be the case by Pert and her colleagues (1973). In the presence of salt, the binding of all agonists is decreased, whereas that of antagonists is enhanced. This discriminatory effect was found only with sodium ions and to a lesser extent with lithium. All other alkali and alkaline earth ions were found to reduce binding of both agonists and antagonists. Simon presented data confirming the

TABLE 9

Effect of Organic and Inorganic Cations on Stereospecific Opiate
Binding to Rat Brain Homogenate [Simon et al., 1975]

Reagent	Final concentra-tion (mM)	Levorphanol binding (% of control)	Naltrexone binding (% of control)
NaCl	200	16	180
	100	22	180
	50	37	160
	5	−	120
	1	−	0
KCl	200	−	70
	100	64	85
Putrescine	100	26	40
	50	−	54
	10	68	−
	5	−	97
	1	75	106
Spermidine	100	1	10
	50	−	32
	10	50	−
	5	−	78
	1	95	−
Choline	100	100	97
Poly-L-Lysine (MW 400,000)	1.25×10^{-4} (50 μg/ml)	46	103

Reagents were added in 0.05 M Tris-HCl, pH 7.4, to 2.0 ml of rat brain P_2 fraction during preincubation with unlabeled levorphanol or dextrorphan (10^{-6} M). The labeled ligand concentrations were: ^{3}H-levorphanol (specific activity: 6 c/mmole) 5×10^{-9} M, ^{3}H-naltrexone (specific activity 15.3 c/mmole) 1×10^{-9} M. ^{3}H-levorphanol incubation mixtures contained 1.7 to 2.3 mg protein/ml and ^{3}H-naltrexone incubation mixtures 0.9 to 1.4 mg protein/ml. Control samples bound stereospecifically an average of 1000 counts/min of ^{3}H-levorphanol and 3750 counts/min of ^{3}H-naltrexone.

uniqueness of sodium. He showed that a number of organic cations are also incapable of discriminating between agonists and antagonists (Table 9).

The question of whether the changes produced by sodium are due to changes in the number of binding sites, in binding affinities, or both was explored by the Simon group (Simon et al., 1975). Figure 12 shows saturation curves for the binding of ^{3}H-naltrexone in the presence and absence of 100 mM NaCl. At low drug concentration, salt enhances naltrexone binding over 2-fold, but as the drug concentration

46

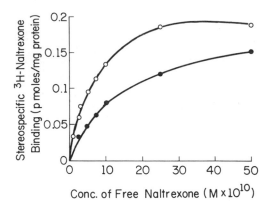

Figure 12. Saturation curves for stereospecific binding of ^{3}H-naltrexone. Rat brain P_2 fraction (1.2 mg protein/ml) was preincubated for 5 min with levorphanol or dextrorphan (10^{-6} M), followed by 15 min incubation with various concentrations of ^{3}H-naltrexone (specific activity 15.3 c/mmole). (●) 0.5 M Tris-HCl, pH 7.4; (○) 0.10 M NaCl in 0.5 M Tris-HCl, pH 7.4. [Simon et al., 1975]

is raised this enhancement becomes smaller and smaller. A Klotz double reciprocal plot of the data, shown in Figure 13, indicates that the lines intersect on the Y-axis. Since the Y-intercept represents the reciprocal of the maximum number of binding sites, there is no difference in the

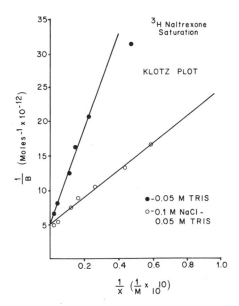

Figure 13. Double reciprocal plot of naltrexone binding. The data presented in Figure 12 are replotted in the manner suggested by Klotz (1950). [Simon et al., 1975]

number of binding sites. Scatchard presentation of the data (not shown) leads to the same conclusion. Thus, the enhancement of naltrexone binding in NaCl is the result of increased affinity (K_D = 5 × 10^{-10} M in salt, 1.1 × 10^{-9} M in sodium-free Tris buffer). There is no evidence for unmasking of new sites, according to Simon.

A similar analysis of the decrease in agonist (etorphine) binding in sodium indicated that here also the major change is one of binding affinity, in the case of etorphine a 5-fold decrease. There is essentially no decrease in the number of binding sites (except at salt concentrations above 200 mM where a nonspecific decrease in binding for both agonists and antagonists is superimposed on the discriminatory effect under discussion). The analysis in the case of etorphine was complicated by the fact that, at the salt concentrations used (100-150 mM), residual sites with affinity characteristic of the salt-free state as well as transformed lower affinity sites (sodium-type) coexist. This gives rise to the S-shaped curve shown in Figure 14. The initial experiments were carried only to the first plateau and gave the erroneous impression of a decrease in binding sites. However, when saturation curves were carried to higher concentrations, it became evident that binding in sodium approached that seen in the absence of sodium. Simon suggested that his data are consistent with the model that opiate receptors exist in (at least) two distinct conformational states, one characteristic of the absence of sodium and the other of the presence of sodium. The

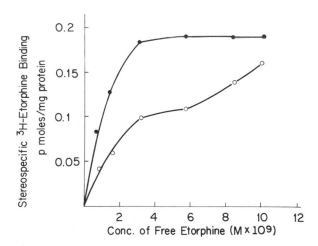

Figure 14. Saturation curves for stereospecific binding of ^{3}H-etorphine. Incubation as described in Figure 12. Protein concentration of P_2 fraction was 1.0 mg/ml. (●) 0.05 M Tris-HCl, pH 7.4; (○) 0.15 M NaCl in 0.05 M Tris-HCl, pH 7.4. [Simon et al., 1975]

sodium-dependent state has a lower affinity for agonists and a greater affinity for antagonists than the sodium-free state. This model is also consistent with the finding in Snyder's and in Simon's laboratories that ED_{50} (effective median dose) concentrations of agonists for competition with labeled antagonists increase in the presence of sodium. Changes in ED_{50} reflect changes in affinity.

Pasternak suggested that apparent alterations in affinity can be explained by changes in the number of the two distinct binding sites. The high-affinity site is the one affected by sodium, with an increase in high-affinity naloxone binding and a decrease in high-affinity dihydromorphine binding. Simon has analyzed his Scatchard and Klotz curves by drawing a single straight line, when, at the concentrations of ^{3}H-opiate Simon uses, he is looking at a mixture of high- and low-affinity sites. Thus, when sodium increases the number of high-affinity sites, it appears as a change in affinity, because the high- and low-affinity sites are not separated. The primary reason the high-affinity site was not more obvious in Simon's experiments, according to Pasternak, is that concentrations of tritiated opiates employed are not sufficiently low.

Simon replied to Pasternak's comments as follows: (1) The naltrexone concentrations used in Simon's laboratory ranged from 0.1 nM (comparable to the lowest concentration of naloxone used by the Snyder group) to 5 nM. The affinity of naltrexone (1 nM in the absence, 0.5 nM in the presence of sodium) is also comparable to that of naloxone (0.6-0.9 nM) to what Snyder termed the high-affinity receptor. Since naloxone has a K_D of 60 nM to the low-affinity receptor and naltrexone presumably a similar one (based on similarity in structure and affinity to high-affinity receptor), the concentration range of naltrexone utilized is well within the high-affinity receptor range, and very few low-affinity receptors should be occupied even at the highest naltrexone concentrations used. (2) The low-affinity receptor was reported by Snyder (this meeting) to be relatively unaffected by the presence of sodium. It is, therefore, difficult to see how it can contribute to the sodium effect when its level of binding remains constant. (3) As reported by both laboratories, log-probit plots of competition for binding of agonists with labeled antagonists are parallel in the presence and absence of sodium. Such parallel lines usually denote a single and identical receptor in the two situations. The ED_{50} changes obtained from these plots are related to changes in affinity, and ED_{50}'s are readily converted to K_D's. (4) In Simon's laboratory, experiments have been carried out to demonstrate that an agonist can displace an antagonist from all its sites, and, conversely, an antagonist can completely displace an agonist, in both the presence and absence of NaCl. These results are inconsistent with the suggestion from Snyder's laboratory that the number of binding sites recognized by antagonists in the presence of sodium is greater than the number recognized by agonists.

In summary, Simon reiterated that all of his data and the bulk of data from Snyder's laboratory favor the simple, parsimonious model he has advanced, in which the same number of receptors exist in two conformational (sodium-dependent and sodium-free) states.

Simon also reported that heating homogenates at 50°C for two minutes increases naltrexone binding even in the presence of 100 mM NaCl (Figure 15). Longer heating resulted in gradual loss of binding capacity. In addition, a dissociation curve for ^{3}H-etorphine was presented that showed two distinct dissociation slopes. Pasternak suggested the two rates might be due to the presence of two affinity binding sites, because the rate of dissociation is closely related to the

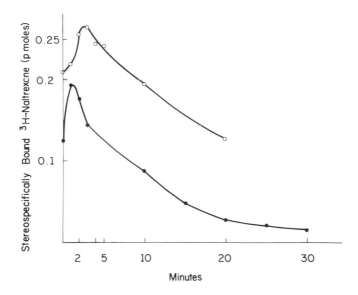

Figure 15. Heat denaturation of ^{3}H-naltrexone binding capacity of rat brain P_2 fraction were equilibrated for 5 min at 37°C and then heated at 50°C for 1 to 30 min. Subsequently ^{3}H-naltrexone (1 × 10^{-9} M) binding was carried out at 37°C as described in Figure 12. P_2 fraction contained 1 mg protein/ml. (●) 0.05 M Tris-HCl, pH 7.4, (○) 0.10 M NaCl in 0.05 M Tris-HCl, pH 7.4. [Simon et al., 1975]

affinity of the receptor for the ligand. Simon replied that, since two distinct slopes for etorphine dissociation are seen only in salt, the second slope (essentially parallel to the slope in Tris buffer) may represent the sites still present in the untransformed, sodium-free form.

Solubilization of an Opiate Binding Component from Mouse Brain: A. Goldstein

Goldstein suggested that there are several opiate binding sites, more than the two described by Pasternak and Snyder (1975). Thus, there may or may not be differences between his opiate binding component and that described by Snyder's, Terenius's, and Simon's groups. The component Goldstein is working with is insoluble in water and in most of the common detergents. Therefore, a procedure similar to that reported by Folch and his co-workers (1957), Mokrasch (1967), and Soto and his colleagues (1969) using a chloroform-methanol extraction was developed.

In his initial attempts to solubilize the receptor, Goldstein washed with water to remove ionic substituents, after which the properties of material remaining in the chloroform-methanol phase were altered. A second washing brings a great deal of material into the interface between water and organic solvent. This interface contains all the stereospecific binding. Proteolipids behave in this fashion, suggesting that the binding material might be a proteolipid. Goldstein subsequently followed the pattern of the opiate binding substance on the Sephadex LH-20 column, which fractionates materials by solubility as well as by molecular sieving. The column is eluted with the least polar solvent, chloroform, then by increased amounts of methanol. De Robertis (1971) has used this technique to study binding substances for a variety of neurotransmitters.

To measure binding of opiates in these fractions, Goldstein employed a technique developed in De Robertis's laboratory involving the partition of the radioactive ligand between an aqueous and an organic solvent. Initial studies showed only nonspecific binding. Results were more promising when ether precipitation was used to remove the bulk of the lipids. The ether precipitate is redissolved, and binding is studied with 0.4 μM radioactive levorphanol. Under these conditions there is no binding in the early fractions, but there is a sharp peak in the 50% chloroform-methanol fraction, which is reduced by nonradioactive levorphanol. Similarly, this peak cannot be demonstrated with radioactive dextrorphan employed in the same experiment with radioactive levorphanol of another label.

In other experiments, varying degrees of stereospecificity were obtained. This suggests that the binding sites are labile and, upon denaturation, change in the degree of their stereospecificity. More reproducible data were obtained using a lipid antioxidant.

The binding function studied by Goldstein has been found only in the brain and in the guinea pig ileum and not in other tissues. It is either saturable or nonsaturable, depending on the concentration range examined. There is saturation in the 0.1 μM range, but then binding increases, followed by another plateau. At much higher concentrations, the binding is not saturable.

After the binding material has reacted with radioactive ligand and has been refractionated on the same column, its properties change, and the peak of radioactivity emerges earlier in a more lipophilic region of the column. This shift is a useful tool in purifying a substance. Because the receptor substance is not dialysable, one can bind a ligand to the "receptor," rechromatograph it, dialyze away the ligand, and reinstitute the purification sequence.

Cerebrosides: H.H. Loh

Loh first emphasized the complementary structure of cerebrosides to opiates. Cerebrosides provide sites for interaction of the benzene ring of opiates with the piperidine ring of opiates. Cerebroside sulfate provides a geometrically ideal anionic site for binding to the amine nitrogen of opiates. Loh observed substantial binding of ^{3}H-naloxone and ^{3}H-etorphine to common commercial preparations of cerebrosides from bovine brain. About 20% of total binding is stereospecific. The commercial preparation contains 4 different compounds: cerebroside, hydroxycerebroside, cerebroside sulfate, and hydroxycerebroside sulfate. About 10% to 15% of the total material is cerebroside sulfate and hydroxycerebroside sulfate.

When saturation curves are made, multiple apparent binding affinities are observed, involving 4 plateaus. The highest affinity binding, which saturates at about 10 nM, involves cerebroside sulfate, another site occurs at 40 nM, and the 2 other sites are of less affinity.

Etorphine has an affinity of 10 nM. Morphine has an affinity of about 5 μM, about the same as levorphanol, while dextrorphan has an affinity of about 1 to 5 mM. Etorphine, therefore, is about 200 times more potent than morphine in displacing radioactive etorphine. With radioactive naloxone, the two drugs differ in affinity only by a factor of 10. With both radioactive etorphine and naloxone, morphine is slightly more potent than levorphanol. The affinity for codeine is 45 μM. The two methadone isomers differ in affinity only by a factor of 2.

Loh attempted to determine the extent to which commercial cerebrosides mimic behavior of the stereospecific binding substance in brain described by Goldstein as a possible opiate receptor. Using the Sephadex LH-20 column it is possible to separate the various cerebrosides. Hydroxy- and nonhydroxy-cerebroside sulfates are eluted in the same fraction as Goldstein's binding substance. Thin-layer chromatography of this fraction reveals a small amount of phosphatidyl serine, which, however, is present to a much greater extent in more lipophilic parts of the membrane. However, the major constituent is cerebroside sulfate. Just as described by Goldstein for his stereospecific binding substance in brain extracts, when cerebroside sulfate is complexed with levorphanol it migrates on the column to a more lipophilic area. Not only does commercial cerebroside sulfate emerge from the column in the same location as the Goldstein receptor, but in brain extracts chemical measurement of cerebroside sulfate reveals it to be primarily in the same fraction.

To determine the apparent amino acid content, material hydrolyzed by 6 N HCl has been analyzed. Fluorescamine-reacting substances are released. However, this can be attributed to nitrogen released from a cerebroside. Using commercially available cerebrosides, Loh has shown that most of the apparent amino nitrogen in the putative opiate receptor of Goldstein can be accounted for by the nitrogen content of cerebroside sulfate.

If cerebroside sulfate binds morphine, what relationship does this have to the pharmacological actions of opiates? Jimpy mice have a low brain content of cerebroside sulfate. These mice are very resistant to the pharmacological actions of morphine, requiring 6 times more morphine to produce analgesia than normal mice. This insensitivity to morphine cannot be accounted for by penetration of morphine into the brain. In these mice the cerebroside sulfate concentration in the brain is only 60% of control mice.

Cuatrecasas raised some of the critical questions in the discrepant results of Loh and Goldstein. Is cerebroside sulfate identical to the presumed proteolipid of Goldstein? Is cerebrosulfatide a pharmacologically relevant opiate receptor? Even if cerebroside sites are not pharmacologically relevant opiate receptors, are there related molecules serving such functions? Is the opiate receptor binding of membrane fractions related at all to the cerebroside sulfate binding?

Goldstein has been able to confirm Loh's findings. Trypsin treatment does not affect the amide bond in cerebrosides. Goldstein calculates that 500 amino groups are released per bound opiate. Cerebrosides contain only one amino group per molecule, so that one would have to argue that one opiate molecule binds to 500 cerebroside molecules. Using molecular models Goldstein does not believe that one could obtain stereospecific binding to a cerebroside. Cuatrecasas pointed out that micelle formation can readily explain the apparent binding of 500 amino groups per opiate molecule.

Loh replied that the most careful amino analysis fails to reveal any protein content. This contradicts Goldstein's assertion that the stereospecific binding could occur only with a protein backbone to the lipid. Moreover, with a very sensitive thin-layer chromatographic analysis that can resolve small amounts of amino acids, none can be demonstrated.

Kosterlitz pointed out that if cerebroside sulfate is related to the pharmacological actions of morphine, its distribution throughout the brain should parallel the localization of pain perception mechanisms and true opiate receptor binding. Cerebroside sulfate content is highest in the brainstem, where Goldstein has described the highest density of opiate binding substance. By contrast, specific opiate receptor binding in synaptic membranes is relatively low in the brainstem (Kuhar et al., 1973). Of course, as Goldstein has suggested, if protein is critical for this binding, then regional distribution of cerebroside would not be a relevant question. Still, Cuatrecasas emphasized that pure cerebroside sulfates do bind opiates stereospecifically, suggesting no need to postulate any protein in this binding substance.

Cuatrecasas pointed to an analogous situation in which cholera toxin binds *very* specifically to ganglioside G_{M1} and subsequently stimulates adenylate cyclase. However, the response at a biological level to cholera toxin does not correlate specifically with the number of G_{M1} molecules in the tissue, principally because the number of G_{M1}

gangliosides is greatly in excess of the number of cyclase molecules in most tissues. Clearly, the biological response also depends on the transduction between the recognition sites and another effector site. The kinetics of the binding is also critical. One can even manipulate the biological response by adding ganglioside molecules to cells. The gangliosides are incorporated into the membrane, and the cell then shows a greater response to cholera toxin. It is now fairly well established that these special glycolipids are the biological receptors for cholera toxin (Cuatrecasas, 1973a,b,d).

Snyder advised caution in ascribing biological significance to binding, even though a few compounds parallel affinity for binding and pharmacological potency. Extensive series of homologous drugs such as the ketobemidones should be evaluated, as has been done successfully for specific opiate receptor binding of synaptic membranes. With regard to the jimpy mice, it is important to evaluate other neurologically mutant mice, because the aberrant response of jimpy mice to morphine may be due to general neurological impairment and not to a selective abnormality in cerebroside sulfates.

An important area for future research is the relevance of the cerebroside sulfate described by Loh to the opiate receptor. Because cerebroside sulfate does bind opiates with high affinity and some correlation with pharmacological potency, it may be related in some way to the opiate receptors. Perhaps, as Iversen suggested, cerebrosides might be prosthetic groups of the opiate receptor, as heme is related to globin in hemoglobin function.

Pasternak observed that opiate binding is extremely sensitive to proteolytic enzymes, but cautioned that they may be solubilizing a protein-cerebroside receptor from membrane. However, he also stated that protein reagents that do not cleave the protein backbone and would not solubilize the proposed protein cerebroside are also extremely effective in destroying stereospecific binding. In addition, the suggestion of the Snyder group that a conformational change is involved with the binding of agonists and antagonists, especially in the presence of sodium chloride, is most easily explained by protein interactions with the binding ligand (Pasternak and Snyder, 1974, 1975; Pasternak et al., 1975; Pert and Snyder, 1974).

Cuatrecasas summarized by explaining that, while it seemed unlikely, the cerebroside could be related to the receptor revealed by stereospecific binding. The only difference between Loh's and

Goldstein's findings is the presence or absence of protein in the solubilized receptor from mouse brain.

Search for the Endogenous Ligand of the Opiate Receptor: J. Hughes

Hughes outlined his reasons for believing that the morphine receptor does not exist by chance and in isolation but in fact forms part of a neurotransmitter or neuromodulator system that functions through the mediation of a naturally occurring "morphine-like" compound, the endogenous ligand. This hypothesis was prompted by the following observations recorded elsewhere in this report: (1) the stereospecific nature of the morphine receptor, (2) the selective distribution of the receptor sites within the brain, and (3) the ability of naloxone to antagonize the analgesic response to focal stimulation of the periaqueductal gray matter.

Hughes adopted a direct approach to testing the hypothesis, simply taking brain extracts and determining whether they exert morphine-like actions. Of course, in any investigation of this sort, great care must be taken to ensure that the observed effects are specifically related to interactions with the opiate receptor. In the mouse vas deferens, inhibition of contractions produced by morphine and other opiates is well correlated with analgesic activity. The mouse vas deferens as a test system was selected for study because it responds to very few compounds, whereas guinea pig ileum contracts and relaxes in response to a multitude of endogenous substances. All opiate actions in the mouse vas deferens are antagonized by low concentrations of naloxone. Therefore, as a critical test for the endogenous ligand, Hughes reasoned that any observed effect should be antagonized by naloxone if it was a specific effect at the opiate receptor.

Starting with 300 g of brain, he extracted with 80% acetone. The resulting homogenate was filtered and the filtrate evaporated; the residues were then dissolved in 30 ml water. Twenty microliters of this produced an effect equivalent to a maximal effect of morphine. Small doses of naloxone (60 nM) partially antagonized this action (Figure 16). When brain extract was again added in the presence of naloxone, only 50% inhibition of contraction was obtained, whereas 90% inhibition was obtained in the absence of naloxone.

56

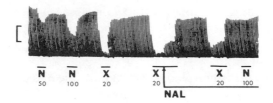

Figure 16. Effect of crude extract from pig brain on neurally evoked contractions of mouse vas deferens. N = normorphine 50 and 100 ng. X = 20 μl extract from 30 ml stock ≡ 300 g brain. Naloxone (60 nM) partially antagonised the effect of the extract. Vertical calibration = 100 mg. [Hughes]

When the mixture was extracted with ethylacetate and ether to remove organic substances, the extract seemed less potent, but naloxone became more effective in reversing its actions. This new extract no longer produced so great an effect in the presence of naloxone.

Using column and thin-layer chromatographic procedures, Hughes has purified this substance to get a white powder that is being analyzed by mass spectrometry. The substance is hydrophilic and does not dissolve in organic solvents such as acetone, ethylacetate, or benzene, but does dissolve in methanol and in water. It is stable toward heating at 80°C for 1 h, light, and acid conditions. There is a single UV absorption peak at 270 nM. The chromatographic properties of the endogenous ligand rule out identity with morphine or other common opiates. Its apparent molecular weight, determined by Sephadex exclusion, is 300 to 700. It does not react with ninhydrin or fluorescamine.

The inhibitory action of the purified extract on electrically evoked twitches of the mouse vas deferens was almost completely abolished by the three narcotic antagonists naloxone (Figure 17), naltrexone, and Mr 1302.

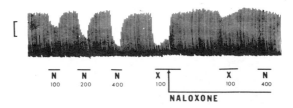

Figure 17. Reversal and antagonism by naloxone (60 nM) of inhibition by purified extract in the mouse vas deferens. N = normorphine, 100, 200 and 400 ng. X = 20 μl of purified extract. Vertical calibration = 100 mg. [Hughes]

The endogenous ligand acted more rapidly than normorphine, and after washing out the bath, its effects were reversed slightly more rapidly than were those of normorphine. With partially purified extracts, Hughes has examined the regional distribution in the rat brain. The partially purified acetone powder had a specific activity in normorphine equivalents of 700-800 µg/mg. Thus, if this material is completely pure, its potency is about the same as that of normorphine. In rabbit brain, normorphine equivalent values for various brain areas were as follows: 0.2-0.4 µg/g in the cerebral cortex; undetectable in the cerebellum; 5-10 µg/g in the corpus striatum; 1-2 µg/g in the pons-medulla; and 0.4 µg/g in the hippocampus. Further experiments have failed to detect morphine-like activity in extracts of lung, heart, or spleen. Very small amounts of the endogenous ligand have been detected in human cerebrospinal fluid.

The complex pharmacological activity of crude brain extracts precluded any assay of the endogenous ligand in the guinea pig ileum. Pure preparations of the endogenous ligand, however, showed morphine-like activity on the guinea pig ileum, and its effects could be reversed by naloxone. However, in the guinea pig ileum, the inhibition of the twitch did not stay at a constant level as it did in the mouse vas deferens, but gradually reversed. Therefore it is quite difficult to study naloxone reversal, although one can clearly show that treating the guinea pig ileum with naloxone alters the activity of the endogenous ligand. In general, the brain extracts were significantly less potent in the guinea pig ileum by a factor of 5 to 10. Since guinea pig ileum extracts abolished the action of the endogenous ligand, Hughes has suggested that the guinea pig ileum contains an enzyme that degrades the endogenous ligand, and he has obtained direct evidence for this assertion. The enzymatic activity that destroyed the endogenous ligand was localized to the high-speed supernatant fraction of the guinea pig ileum homogenate.

Further studies on the nature of the endogenous ligand have been carried out by Hughes. Recent work confirms that the material is stable towards trypsin and chymotrypsin but is rapidly destroyed by carboxypeptidase-A and less rapidly by leucine aminopeptidase. The compound therefore is quite unlike any known narcotic analgesic and may be a small peptide with either secondary or tertiary amino groupings.

Binding assays have also been used in the search for endogenous ligands. Terenius described the properties of an apparent endogenous ligand he has isolated (see above, "Narcotic Receptors in Guinea Pig Ileum and Rat Brain"). Pasternak also described a substance in rat brain homogenates that is heat stable and inhibits ^{3}H-naloxone binding. Further studies indicate that this substance closely resembles the endogenous morphine-like substance described by Hughes and Kosterlitz. In rat and calf brain, Pasternak and Snyder found that levels were lowest in the cerebellum, highest in the corpus striatum and hypothalamus, and intermediate in the cerebral cortex. Like Hughes and Kosterlitz, Pasternak and Snyder found that the material is destroyed by carboxypeptidase-A but is affected much less by trypsin and chymotrypsin and is stable to boiling. Because the apparent endogenous ligand inhibits ^{3}H-naloxone binding less in the presence of sodium, it behaves like an opiate agonist, again agreeing with Hughes and Kosterlitz. While sodium selectively decreases opiate agonist binding, Pasternak and Snyder recently noted that low concentrations of manganese selectively increase agonist binding with little influence on antagonists. Their observation that manganese enhances endogenous ligand-induced decreases in ^{3}H-naloxone binding indicates further the agonist character of the endogenous ligand. In the experiments of Pasternak and Snyder, the endogenous ligand does not pass through dialysis tubing and is excluded on a Biogel P-2 column, indicating a molecular weight of 2,000 or more. In addition, the material passes through several Amicon filters with molecular weight cutoff values of 10,000, indicating that its molecular weight is less than 10,000.

III. AGONIST-ANTAGONIST INTERACTIONS

Introduction

Opiate agonist-antagonists such as nalorphine can relieve pain because of their agonist properties and can produce physical dependence but not drug craving or psychological dependence. Thus they offer potential as relatively nonaddicting analgesics, and they have stimulated much clinical interest. Attempts were made to use nalorphine as an analgesic, but patients could not tolerate its unpleasant psychotomimetic and sedative-hypnotic effects. Nalorphine's agonist properties, however, stimulated the massive screening of opiate antagonists in the hope of discovering a nonaddicting analgesic. A number of drugs have emerged from this effort. Some, like profadol and propiram, have pure opiate-like agonist activity and seem to be morphine agonists with less intrinsic activity than morphine (Jasinski et al., 1971). They produce morphine-like agonist activity in single doses and morphine-like physical dependence when chronically administered. However, in subjects dependent on large amounts of morphine, they precipitate abstinence because of their lower intrinsic activity. In subjects dependent on smaller amounts of morphine, these compounds suppress abstinence. Because of these properties they are termed "partial agonists" (Table 10). Profadol and propiram have not been promoted for clinical use. By contrast, agonist-antagonists of the benzomorphan series include agents that have been used extensively in man as analgesics.

Pentazocine (Talwin) is the most widely employed benzomorphan analgesic. Pentazocine produces effects common to both the opiate prototype, morphine, and the opiate antagonist, nalorphine. In doses from 20 to 40 mg, it produces subjective effects in humans similar to 5 to 10 mg of morphine. At higher dose levels, about 60 to 70 mg, pentazocine produces dysphoric sedative-hypnotic and psychotomimetic effects comparable to those seen with nalorphine. Unlike nalorphine, pentazocine can elicit significant analgesia at dose levels that do not give rise to the sedative-hypnotic or psychotomimetic effects of nalorphine. Like nalorphine, however, pentazocine can precipitate abstinence in subjects dependent on 240 mg of morphine/day. Pentazocine is 1/50 as potent as nalorphine as an opiate antagonist.

TABLE 10

Opiate Agonists, Antagonists, and Agonist-Antagonists
[Mansky, from data of Martin and Jasinski, Addiction Research Center]

Opiate	Subjective effect (single dose)		Physical dependence (withdrawal syndrome)		Morphine antagonist		Drug dependence (drug craving upon withdrawal)
	Morphine-like euphoria	Nalorphine-like dysphoria	Morphine-like	Nalorphine-like	Low habit (60 mg morphine/day)	High habit (240 mg morphine/day)	
Agonist							
Morphine							
Heroin							
Codeine	yes	no	yes	no	no	no	yes
Meperidine							
Methadone							
Dextropropoxyphene							
Agonist-antagonist							
Nalorphine	yes	yes	no	yes	yes	yes	no
"Pure" antagonist							
Naloxone	no	no	no	no	yes	yes	no
Partial agonist							
Propiram							
Profadol	yes	no	yes	no	no	yes	yes
Pentazocine	yes	yes	yes	yes	no data	yes	yes

With chronic administration, tolerance and dependence develop to pentazocine. Withdrawal of pentazocine after chronic administration of the drug leads to an abstinence syndrome that shows similarities to both the morphine and the nalorphine abstinence syndromes. The abstinence syndromes of pentazocine, nalorphine, and morphine can be distinguished by rank ordering the physiological parameters (see Chapter VI, "Addiction"). Pentazocine appears to produce a syndrome that shares the qualities of both morphine and nalorphine syndromes. Unlike nalorphine but like morphine, withdrawal from pentazocine leads to prominent drug-seeking behavior (Jasinski et al., 1970) (see Table 10).

The opiate agonist-antagonists have also been used in the treatment of opiate dependence. Nonaddicted opiate users have been administered cyclazocine on a chronic basis, with tolerance developing to the physiological and subjective effects of this drug. Tolerance does not develop to the ability of cyclazocine to antagonize the agonist actions of morphine or heroin (Martin et al., 1966). Thus, well-motivated opiate users have been able to remain nonopiate dependent with the chronic administration of cyclazocine. Naloxone and naltrexone (Martin et al., 1973c) have also been used in this type of treatment.

Chemical Components of Agonism and Antagonism:
A.E. Jacobson

The basic opiate-analgesic structure involves a phenolic ring attached to a carbon that has no hydrogen substitutions and that, in turn, is attached to a nitrogen through a two-carbon bridge (see Figure 1). Most agonists have a methyl substitution on the nitrogen, whereas most antagonists possess N-allyl, N-cyclopropylmethyl, or N-propyl groups. N-allyl norcodeine was the first known antagonist, synthesized by Pohl in 1915. Nalorphine was the first well-recognized antagonist, and it was found to possess agonist activity. Gates and Montzka (1964) introduced the N-cyclopropylmethyl group on analgesics because it is electronically similar to allyl groups, and, in fact, it confers stronger antagonist properties than N-allyl on appropriate molecules.

Among the morphinans, levallorphan is the most prominent antagonist and also possesses some agonist properties. Some of the most interesting agonist-antagonists are derived from the benzomorphans.

Metazocine and phenazocine are pure agonists, while pentazocine is a mixed, relatively weak agonist-antagonist. The mixed, strong agonist-antagonists generally possess psychotomimetic side effects.

Substituting a hydroxyl group on the 14-position in morphine-like molecules or on the 9-position of benzomorphans may change the pharmacological characteristics of the compound. In general, this hydroxyl group, when in a position to hydrogen bond to the nitrogen, gives much purer N-substituted antagonists. An example is the agonist oxymorphone and the corresponding "pure" antagonists, naloxone (N-allyl) and naltrexone (N-cyclopropylmethyl).

The oripavine series of compounds provides the most potent known opiates. These molecules have six rings. The rationale behind their design was to provide more rigid and complex molecules that, with their stringent structural requirements, could fit selectively into the receptor. When the N-substituent is cyclopropylmethyl, diprenorphine, a pure antagonist, is obtained; whereas buprenorphine, with a different C-7 side chain, is a mixed agonist-antagonist.

The bicyclic and monocyclic opiates, those based on the phenylmorphans and ketobemidones, are more complex in that the usual molecular manipulations required to confer antagonist properties do not succeed with these analgesics. The common N-substituents (allyl, cyclopropylmethyl, etc.) do not confer antagonist properties on these molecules. It may be of interest to note, however, that replacement of methyl on the nitrogen atom of ketobemidone by amyl, hexyl, or heptyl does produce good agonists with long-lasting, nalorphine-like properties in morphine-dependent monkeys, although of lower potency than nalorphine. For the ketobemidones (from methyl to decyl on the nitrogen atom of ketobemidone, prepared by T. Oh-ishi, R. Wilson, and M. Rogers in Jacobson's laboratory), in vitro receptor binding affinities measured by Pert and Snyder (Wilson et al., 1975b) are in good agreement with in vivo agonist activity. This evidence of good correlation between in vitro receptor affinity and in vivo agonist activity is not, by any means, inevitably found. For example, with the 9-α and 9-β series of benzomorphans, this correlation was not found in work done by Klee.* The 9-α series consists of molecules in which the substituent at the 9-position is oriented away from the nitrogen atom. The 9-β benzomorphans have substituents that sterically block the nitrogen atom to electrophilic attack, and some of

*W. Klee, personal communication.

these have agonist activity an order of magnitude greater than the comparable compounds in the 9-α series. The in vitro receptor binding affinities for the 9-α vs the 9-β compounds only occasionally correlate with their in vivo activity. Due to this occasional correlation, it is difficult to fit transport into the picture as an added parameter.

The picture of the narcotic receptor that emerges from these data is complex. Certainly the "receptor," assuming there is but one type of receptor for analgesia, must be quite flexible. It accepts morphine, which has a fixed axially oriented aromatic group and a B-C *cis* ring junction, rejects the *trans* (B-C) morphine, but will accept both the B-C *cis* and *trans* morphinan and the more or less freely rotating, equatorially oriented aromatic ring in pethidine-like molecules and phenylmorphans.

Returning to the monocyclic type of agonist, it is noteworthy that pethidine and methadone agonists have not been converted into antagonists. Moreover, no one has attempted to convert the powerful benzimidazole agonist, etonitazine, to an antagonist (Figure 18). Weak

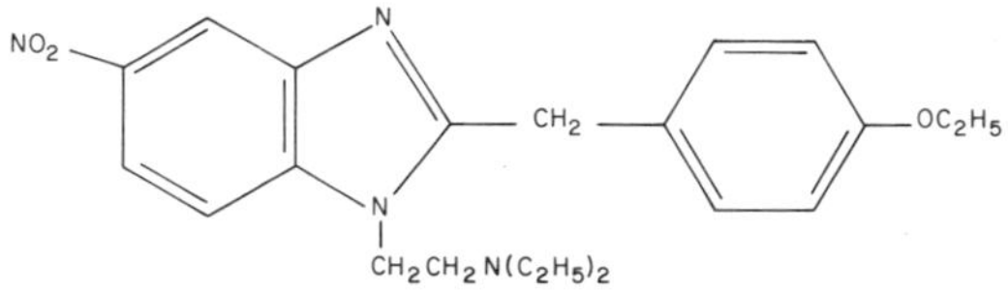

Figure 18. Structure of etonitazine. [Jacobson]

antagonists have been prepared from β-pethidine (N-allyl), which has the phenyl and carbethoxy groups in the 3- rather than 4-position (Figure 19). This compound lends support to the hypothesis of Archer and his co-workers (1964) that a β-phenethylamine fragment is a structural prerequisite for antagonism. More than likely, however, it is more complex than that simple statement would indicate.

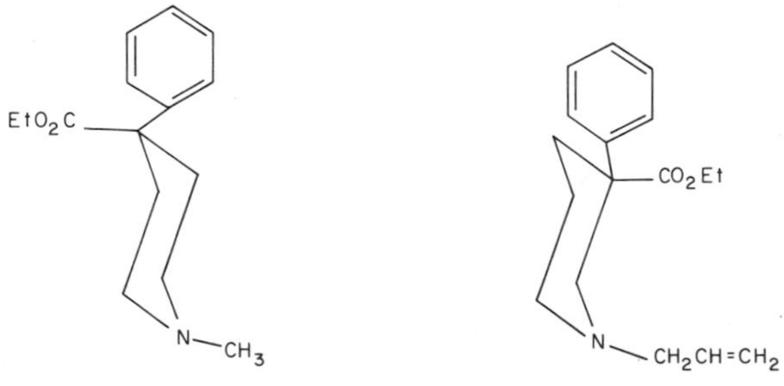

Figure 19. Structure of pethidine (*left*) and N-allylnor-β-pethidine (*right*). [Jacobson]

Lastly, it is interesting to note that certain optical isomers in the N-methyl benzomorphan series appear to be typical nalorphine-like antagonists in physically dependent monkeys. N-methyl levo-isomers in the profadol and phenylmorphan series also appear to be antagonists in mouse and monkey species. Thus, evidently N-methyl antagonists can also be prepared. Former theories relating to the necessity for a 3-carbon chain on nitrogen to promote antagonism are now regarded as rather doubtful. In fact, except for the tricyclic to hexacyclic compounds with the well-known allyl, cyclopropylmethyl, etc., groups on nitrogen, it is difficult for a chemist to predict, a priori, whether a new compound will prove to be an antagonist. It is much simpler to predict the in vivo analgesic activity of, at least, the benzomorphans from their molecular structure, using recently completed work from Jacobson's laboratory involving the Hansch method of analysis (Jacobson, 1975).

Jacobson concluded this review of a number of the known antagonists, based on the monocyclic to hexacyclic molecular structures of the parent agonist, by noting that predictions, a priori, of antagonist activity from molecular structure are difficult to impossible on all but the well-trodden paths. Affinities of the parent agonists for in vitro receptor preparations do occasionally accord with in vivo determined analgesic activity of these compounds. Pert and Snyder's (1974) in vitro receptor work, using the sodium:no-sodium ratio, appears to be fairly successful in distinguishing agonist and antagonist activities, as is Kosterlitz's guinea pig ileum method (Kosterlitz et al., 1973a,b; Kosterlitz and Waterfield, 1975). Jacobson noted, however, a few compounds that appear to contradict the data of Pert and Snyder (1974), in that they are predicted to be antagonists by their sodium: no-sodium ratio, but in vivo monkey studies show they are not. The issue of a single type of analgesic "receptor" vs closely allied dual, or perhaps multiple, "receptors" is difficult to resolve from these data.

To recapitulate some of the known data concerning the antagonists:

1. Given an aromatic hydroxyl group in the *meta*-position to a quaternary, or in some instances, tertiary carbon atom in tricyclic to hexacyclic structures, strong agonists (6,7-benzomorphans, morphinans, morphines, and endo-ethenyloripavines) can be converted to commensurately strong antagonists by replacement of methyl on nitrogen by allyl, propyl, or cyclopropylmethyl as the preferred groups. In all of

these cases, the benzene ring is in fixed axial position, and there is a phenethylamine arrangement in the molecule.

2. When the group on nitrogen is cyclobutylmethyl, agonist properties markedly predominate over antagonist properties.

3. A 14-hydroxyl group in the morphinans and morphine and the corresponding 9-hydroxyl group in 6,7-benzomorphans appear to be favorable for inducing nearly pure antagonist action.

4. The strong phenylmorphan (bicyclic structures) and (mono-cyclic) ketobemidone agonists, each with a nonrigid equatorial *meta*-hydroxyphenyl residue but without a phenethylamine system, do not give antagonists by the usual N-substitution. However, replacement of methyl on nitrogen of ketobemidone with amyl, hexyl, or heptyl produces strong agonists that also have nalorphine-like properties of long duration as judged by their effects on the morphine-dependent monkey.

5. Methadone and pethidine, with none of the structural features cited previously, do not give antagonists. N-Allylnor-β-pethidine (with a phenethylamine moiety) is a very weak antagonist.

6. Some (−)-isomers in the N-methyl-benzomorphan, phenyl-morphan, and profadol series are nalorphine-like antagonists in the very sensitive test in morphine-dependent monkeys.

Opiate Antagonism in Vivo: A.E. Takemori

Usually the concept of pA_x (Schild, 1957) is used with isolated tissue preparations to identify agonists acting on similar receptors. Takemori's group has in recent years applied the concept of pA_x in intact animals to the characterization of analgesic receptors. The definition of the apparent pA_2 in vivo then becomes the negative logarithm of the molar dose of the injected antagonist that reduces the effect of a double dose of an agonist to that of a single dose. The concentration of the antagonist at the receptor site is unknown, but it is assumed to be proportional to the dose.

Although pA_2 is regarded as equal to the log of the affinity constant (K_B) of the antagonist for the receptor, this is not entirely true in vivo. However, the "K_B" in vivo should be proportional to the real K_B if the above assumption about the antagonist concentration is correct.

Aside from the theoretical implications of "pA_2" in vivo, the procedure offers a means to summarize a large amount of quantitative data on competitive drug antagonism and a standard method to compare antagonists. Takemori's group has used this procedure for the characterization of receptors interacting with agonist and antagonist analgesics to compare the type of narcotic-receptor interaction involved in various analgesic assays and to compare potencies of certain narcotic antagonists (Takemori, 1973). The concept of pA_x has also been used to gather evidence that morphine causes a structural change in analgesic receptors. In studies in vivo, the agonists morphine, levorphanol, and methadone generate the same pA_2 as naloxone of 7, indicating that they act at the same site, whereas the mixed agonist-antagonists pentazocine, cyclazocine, and nalorphine have pA_2 values of 6.4. There are either two populations of receptors or one population that responds in different ways to various drugs.

Animals pretreated with morphine were twice as sensitive to naloxone compared to untreated controls (Takemori et al., 1973). This was demonstrated by pretreating mice with a greater than ED_{99} dose of morphine hydrochloride. After 2 hours, at which time the analgesic effect of morphine was no longer evident, dose-response curves for morphine in the absence or presence of 3 increasing doses of naloxone were determined. There was no change in the dose-response curve to morphine alone. However, naloxone caused parallel shifts of the dose-response curve to the right. The same doses of naloxone shifted the dose-response curve substantially more to the right when morphine-pretreated mice were used. This increased sensitivity to naloxone can be computed as a change in the pA_2 value from 6.96 to 7.30. There appeared to be a qualitative change in receptors and the K_B more than doubled from 9.12×10^6 to 2.0×10^7 liters/mole. Takemori interprets this finding to mean that morphine causes a structural change in the analgesic receptors such that the affinity of the receptors for narcotic antagonists is increased. The increased sensitivity to naloxone occurred within 2 hours after a single dose of morphine. In a Japanese strain of mice, this increased sensitivity lasted 3 days, while in American mice the effect lasted only 12 to 24 hours. These discrepancies might be related to the greater sensitivity of Japanese mice to opiates.

The increased sensitivity to naloxone was elicited by all agonists but not by the inactive opiate dextrorphan and not by any mixed agonist-antagonist, such as pentazocine, nor by naloxone itself

(Tulunay and Takemori, 1974a). Morphine pretreatment did not alter the efficacy of naloxone to antagonize the analgesic effect of pentazocine. The increased sensitivity to antagonists can also be obtained when one uses nalorphine or diprenorphine as antagonists instead of naloxone.

These findings suggest the possibility of using this measure as a sensitive indicator of the development of opiate tolerance and physical dependence. Increased sensitivity to naloxone does precede analgesic tolerance, and the potencies of antagonists rise much faster than the development of tolerance. Thereafter, there is a close parallelism of the development of tolerance and enhanced sensitivity to naloxone. When drug administration is terminated, the fall in tolerance and in naloxone sensitivity go hand in hand (Tulunay and Takemori, 1974b).

This change in the apparent affinity constant of the receptors for the antagonist suggests that a qualitative change has taken place in the analgesic receptors with the development of narcotic tolerance. The change is initiated by a single exposure to narcotic drugs, and the receptors continue to change as long as narcotic drugs are available in the milieu. The alteration in receptors stabilizes when the animals become highly tolerant to narcotic drugs.

Takemori feels that the present observations argue against theories of tolerance that infer decreases in the number of pharmacological receptors or increases in the number of silent receptors (Collier, 1966; Castles et al., 1972). If the change in receptors due to narcotic tolerance were a quantitative rather than a qualitative one, the apparent pA_2 value in tolerant animals should have remained the same as that in control animals.

Snyder stated that because increased sensitivity to naloxone is classically associated with physical dependence, the observations of Takemori may reflect a very early state in physical dependence. Moreover, they support the close association of tolerance and physical dependence in terms of basic mechanisms involved.

Cuatrecasas wondered whether Takemori's phenomena might be related to the increased number of receptor binding sites obtained by Pert and Snyder after in vivo administration of morphine (Pert et al., 1973). However, the latter effect occurs at extremely rapid time intervals, as little as 10 min after injection of a drug. Moreover, antagonists produce an increased number of receptor binding sites in much lower doses than are required for opiate agonists

Opiate Actions in Guinea Pig Ileum and Mouse Vas Deferens: H.W. Kosterlitz

In his introductory remarks, Goldstein emphasized that the discovery of isolated in vitro systems has made possible our present understanding of opiate structure-activity relationships. Kosterlitz pointed out that, in vivo, the more lipophilic analog may appear to be the more potent. Metabolic transformations in the liver must also be taken into account; the demethylation of codeine, for example, is mainly responsible for its activity in vivo (Adler, 1963). In isolated systems these factors are largely eliminated.

Kosterlitz emphasized the remarkably close correlation between the inhibitory effects of opiates on the electrically induced contractions of the guinea pig ileum and their ability to relieve pain in man (Kosterlitz et al., 1973a,b) (Figure 20). In addition, the relative

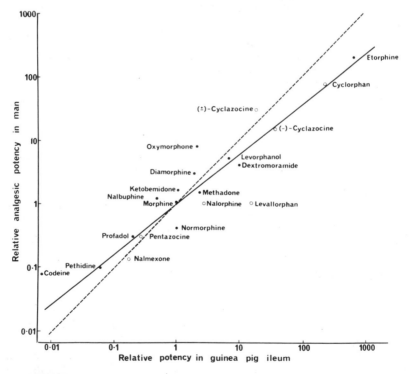

Figure 20. Correlation between the relative agonist potencies of narcotic analgesic drugs in the guinea pig ileum and in analgesia in man (morphine = 1). The values are plotted on a logarithmic scale. Compounds with (○) and without (●) antagonist activity. The sources of the values are given in Kosterlitz and Waterfield (1975). [Kosterlitz]

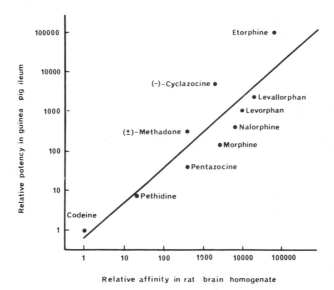

Figure 21. Correlation between the relative potencies to reduce stereospecific binding of ^{3}H-naloxone in rat brain homogenates (no Na[+]) and the relative agonist potencies in the guinea pig ileum (codeine = 1). The values are plotted on a logarithmic scale. Sources of values: Kosterlitz and Watt (1968); Kosterlitz et al. (1973a,b); Kosterlitz and Waterfield (1975); Pert and Snyder (1973b). [Kosterlitz]

potencies of opiate antagonists, as measured by determining their dissociation equilibrium constants, correlate very well (r = 0.986) with their potencies to reduce stereospecific binding in brain homogenates as reported by Pert and Snyder (1973b). The dissociation equilibrium constant cannot be determined in agonists with little antagonist activity. Therefore, the relative potencies of these compounds have been calculated from the concentrations giving a 50% depression of the evoked contraction of the longitudinal muscle of the guinea pig ileum and the values causing a 50% reduction in stereospecific binding in brain homogenates. The correlation (r = 0.905) between relative potencies obtained by the two methods is surprisingly good in spite of the fact that the species, tissues, and experimental procedures were different (Figure 21).

Another smooth muscle system that predicts analgesic potency is the mouse vas deferens; the depression of the contractions elicited by electrical field stimulation is stereospecific and reversed by the antagonists, naloxone and naltrexone. Kosterlitz pointed out that in the guinea pig ileum morphine acts by decreasing the output of acetylcholine, whereas in the mouse vas deferens it acts by decreasing the

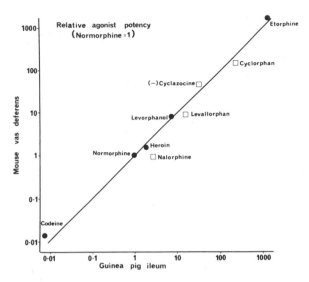

Figure 22. Correlation between the relative potencies of narcotic analgesic drugs in the guinea pig ileum and the mouse vas deferens (normorphine = 1). The values are plotted on a logarithmic scale. Compounds with (□) and without (●) antagonist action. Sources of values: Hughes et al. (1974); Kosterlitz and Watt (1968); Kosterlitz et al. (1973a,b); Kosterlitz and Waterfield (1975); unpublished observations. [Kosterlitz]

output of norepinephrine. The relative potencies of narcotic analgesics obtained in the guinea pig ileum correlate closely with relative potencies in the mouse vas deferens (r = 0.979) (Figure 22). However, when considering absolute values, the vas deferens is some 6 times less sensitive than the guinea pig ileum for compounds with either agonist or antagonist action. Agonist activities of drugs with dual agonist and antagonist activity are more difficult to determine, because these compounds give horizontal dose-response curves. Therefore, for the determination of the agonist action of these drugs, the lowest concentration that gives a depression of the electrically induced contraction has been used (Figure 22). This difference in the relative sensitivities of the two preparations to agonist and antagonist action is probably the basis of the observation that the agonist actions of a mixture of normorphine and nalorphine are additive in the guinea pig ileum, whereas in the mouse vas deferens nalorphine antagonizes the agonist action of normorphine (Figure 23).

Kosterlitz stressed that for the evaluation of the mode of action of new drugs it is important to assess their potencies by all three models, the guinea pig ileum, the mouse vas deferens, and the stereospecific binding in brain homogenates. If discrepancies between

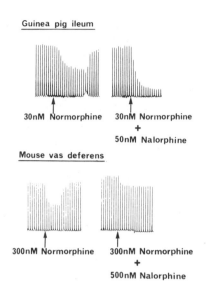

Figure 23. Comparison of the effects of mixtures of normorphine and nalorphine in a segment of guinea pig ileum and in the mouse vas deferens. [Kosterlitz]

the models should arise, it would be likely that the mechanism of action would differ from the drugs examined so far. Such a possibility has been suggested by the findings on a group of compounds that have become available recently. The compounds, N-methylfurylnorcyclazocines and 8-oxocyclazocines, given in Table 11 are all agonists in the guinea pig ileum and the mouse vas deferens and have antinociceptive activity in the writhing and Nilsen tests (Villarreal and Seevers, 1972; Kosterlitz et al., 1973b; Swain and Seevers, 1974*). They have either

TABLE 11

Relative Agonist Potencies [Kosterlitz, Leslie, and Waterfield]

Compound	Guinea pig ileum	Mouse vas deferens	Mouse vas deferens/ guinea pig ileum
Normorphine	1.0	1.0	1.0
2-Methyl-3-methylfuryl- norcyclazocine	1.49 ± 0.15	0.34 ± 0.05	0.23
3-Methylfurylnorcyclazocine	5.6 ± 0.5	1.54 ± 0.10	0.28
8-Oxocyclazocine	68.5 ± 4.3	16.3 ± 1.1	0.24
8-Oxo-5-ethylcyclazocine	397 ± 43	99 ± 11	0.25

The values are the means ± SE of 6 to 9 experiments. The oxo-compounds are the (−)-isomers.

*Also S. Archer and A.K. Pierson, personal communication (1972) and H.W. Kosterlitz, unpublished observations.

no, or only negligible, antagonist activity. Although they are medium to strong agonists, they do not substitute for morphine in the dependent monkey; on the other hand, they do not cause a withdrawal syndrome (Villarreal and Seevers, 1972; Swain and Seevers, 1974). A surprising observation is the finding that, when their agonist activity is compared to normorphine as standard of reference, it is lower in the mouse vas deferens than in the guinea pig ileum (Table 11). If observations in man confirm the results in the dependent monkey that these compounds do not substitute for morphine, it must be concluded that their mode of action differs from morphine and related compounds. The difference between the guinea pig ileum and mouse vas deferens would support this view, although no pharmacological explanation can as yet be offered for this discrepancy.

What might be the anatomical substrate for the endogenous ligand? Elecron micrographs by Gabella (1972) demonstrate four types of terminals. In the guinea pig ileum, no cholinergic fibers enter the longitudinal muscle. Cholinergic terminals, containing characteristic vesicles, lie at the border of the myenteric plexus opposite the muscle. Other terminals face the muscle but contain flat vesicles. Their transmitter content is unknown, but Kosterlitz suggested they might be noradrenergic. There are also typical adrenergic terminals with dense-core vesicles synapsing on the soma. A fourth type of terminal is heterogeneous and contains large granular structures in addition to small clear vesicles. These synapse upon dendrites. There are no transitional states between the large, granular and the small, clear vesicles; the latter strikingly resemble cholinergic vesicles (Figure 24).

Kosterlitz speculated that the endogenous substrate might possibly be localized in the large vesicles. Goldstein felt the terminals with large vesicles resemble those demonstrated by Gershon using autoradiography with radioactive serotonin (Gershon and Altman, 1971). Bloom also felt that Gershon's data are conclusive in showing that the radioactive serotonin is not in a catecholamine terminal, because ^{3}H-5-HT labeling is not eliminated by doses of 6-hydroxydopamine, which do eliminate small, dense-core vesicles that are known to be catecholamine containing. He pointed out that the heterogeneity was an insufficient criterion on which to base the hypothesis that these large granular vesicles produced the endogenous ligand, especially because much evidence did in fact indicate that they were serotonergic. Bloom also pointed out that the terminals resemble the purinergic terminals observed by Burnstock (1972) in the toad intestine.

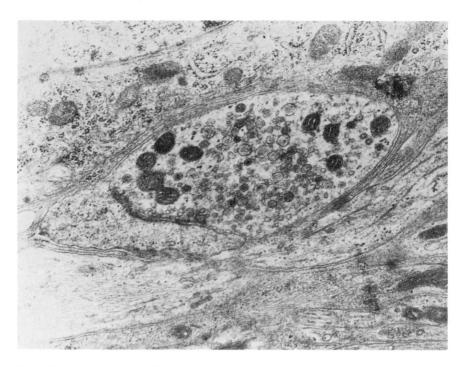

Figure 24. Electron micrograph of myenteric plexus of guinea pig ileum. A nerve process with agranular vesicles and heterogeneous granulated vesicles. Typically, only agranular vesicles are present in the immediate presynaptic area. × 24,000. [Courtesy G. Gabella]

Differential Interactions of Agonists and Antagonists with the Opiate Receptor: C.B. Pert and S.H. Snyder

Pert pointed out that any attempt to explain opiate pharmacology on a molecular basis must grapple with a number of perplexing facts. In contrast to other known systems, opiate agonists and antagonists have strikingly similar structures (Figure 3). Minor chemical modification of opiates results in dramatic shifts in relative agonist-antagonist properties. Even more dramatic is the difference in absolute potency when an opiate antagonist is compared to its corresponding, structurally analogous agonist (see Figure 3). When such agonist/antagonist pairs compete, antagonists are found to be many times more potent in blocking analgesia than agonists are in producing analgesia. On a molecule-for-molecule basis, nalorphine is 200 times more potent than morphine (Grumbach and Chernov, 1965) and cyclazocine is

100 times more potent than phenazocine (Pierson, 1973), to cite two examples. Yet in pharmacological experiments like these, agonists and antagonists generally appear to compete for the same receptors (Takemori et al., 1973).

After a method for biochemically measuring binding to specific opiate receptor sites had been developed, Pert and Snyder (1973a,b) found that opiate agonists, antagonists, and mixed agonist-antagonists all appear to compete for the same receptors in vitro (Pert et al., 1975). Snyder's group hoped that a careful comparison of the binding of radiolabeled opiate agonists with analogous radiolabeled antagonists would reveal differences that would account for their pharmacological actions in vivo.

The concentration of sodium ion in the medium proved to be the critical variable that differentiated agonist from antagonist binding (Pert et al., 1973). The binding of ^{3}H-agonists was invariably decreased by sodium, whereas ^{3}H-antagonist binding was increased (Figure 25). These effects of sodium were exerted at low concentrations; as little as 1 mM sodium ion increased ^{3}H-naloxone binding by 60% while diminishing ^{3}H-dihydromorphine binding by 30%. The effect of sodium is highly specific and not simply the result of alterations in ionic

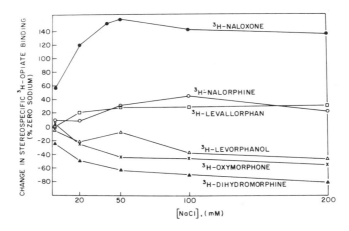

Figure 25. The effect of sodium chloride on the stereospecific binding of 3 ^{3}H-opiate agonists and 3 ^{3}H-opiate antagonists. Each ^{3}H-opiate was incubated in the presence of levallorphan (100 nM) and "dextrallorphan" (100 nM), with varying concentrations of sodium chloride and standard rat brain homogenate that had been "washed" twice. ^{3}H-Naloxone (1 nM), ^{3}H-nalorphine (4 nM), ^{3}H-levallorphan (8.6 nM), ^{3}H-levorphanol (6 nM), ^{3}H-oxymorphone (40 nM), and ^{3}H-dihydromorphine (1 nM), when incubated at 25°C for 30 min in the standard binding assay, gave the following stereospecific control (zero sodium) values respectively: 1292 ± 115 counts/min, 355 ± 30 counts/min, 2170 ± 195 counts/min, 1023 ± 95 counts/min, 694 ± 51 counts/min, and 2570 ± 141 counts/min. [Pert and Snyder, 1974]

strength, because the other monovalent cations examined (potassium, cesium, and rubidium) did not discriminate between agonists and antagonists. Like the divalent cations examined, they merely inhibited binding of both agonists and antagonists at relatively high concentrations (Pert and Snyder, 1974). Only lithium, whose hydration radius is similar to that of sodium, could mimic sodium, although at somewhat higher concentrations.

To further test the generality of "the sodium effect," a method for assessing nonradioactive opiates was devised. The ability of drugs to inhibit ^{3}H-naloxone binding in the absence of sodium was compared to their inhibitory potency in the presence of sodium to obtain a "sodium response ratio" (Figure 26). When a large number of opiates were thus

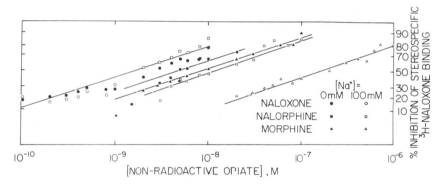

Figure 26. Log-probit analysis of inhibition of stereospecific ^{3}H-naloxone binding in the absence and presence of sodium by nonradioactive naloxone, nalorphine and morphine. ^{3}H-naloxone (1.5 nM) was incubated with standard aliquots of rat brain homogenate and 15 concentrations of nonradioactive drug in triplicate for 30 min at 25°C in the absence and presence of 100 mM NaCl. Control incubations that contained nonradioactive levallorphan (100 nM) or "dextrallorphan" (100 nM) yielded stereospecific binding values of 1479 ± 121 and 3140 ± 300 counts/min in the absence and presence of sodium respectively. [Pert and Snyder, 1974]

examined, their sodium response ratios varied over a very wide range (Figure 27). This ratio appeared to correlate impressively with the pharmacological properties of each drug in vivo: Opiate agonists suffered large losses in inhibitory potency (12- to 60-fold) when sodium was added to the medium. By contrast, "pure" opiate antagonists had response ratios of 1. The potencies of the narcotic antagonists levallorphan, cyclazocine, and nalorphine, which are slightly contaminated by agonist properties in some test situations, were decreased 1.7- to 2.7-fold by sodium. Finally, an intermediate sodium response ratio (3 to 7) was obtained with the mixed agonist-antagonists of the benzomorphan group (Pert et al., 1975).

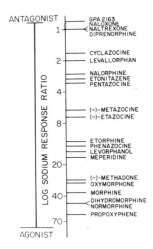

Figure 27. Sodium sensitivity of a number of nonradioactive opiates. The concentration of opiate required to give 50% inhibition of ^{3}H-naloxone binding (1.5 nM) in the presence of 100 mM sodium chloride is divided by the ED_{50} obtained in the absence of sodium to obtain the "sodium response ratio." [C. Pert]

Thus the sodium response ratio seems to be a powerful predictor of the often unpredictable in vivo pharmacological properties of opiates. This is particularly well illustrated in Table 12. It is fascinating that the sodium response ratio varies so greatly within a class of drugs that are usually lumped together as "agonists." Pert speculated that some agonists may be "purer" than others. (Are drugs with higher sodium response ratios more addictive? Are they more effective pain relievers?) On the other end of the spectrum, the experimental 5-phenyl-benzomorphan antagonist GPA 2163 (Clarke et al., 1973) showed a sodium response ratio of *less* than one, suggesting that it may be a purer antagonist than naloxone. It is unclear what pharmacological effects could be produced by a "superpure" antagonist (more intense abstinence precipitation?).

Pert asked how the "sodium effect" works and why it is such a good predictor of relative agonist-antagonist properties in vivo. Double-reciprocal analysis indicates that sodium increases the number of antagonist binding sites while concurrently decreasing the number of agonist binding sites (Pasternak and Snyder, 1974; Pert and Snyder, 1974). Maximal number of binding sites, whether measured with labeled agonist or antagonist, are the same (Creese and Snyder, 1975; Pert and Snyder, 1974). These findings, along with the marked temperature dependence of binding, suggest that the opiate receptor

TABLE 12

Receptor Affinities of Opiates as Influenced by Sodium
[from Pert and Snyder, 1974; Pert et al., 1975]

Drug	Relative affinity for opiate receptor binding* (nM)		Sodium response ratio for opiate receptor binding†
	No sodium	100 mM sodium	
Pure antagonists			
Naloxone	1.5	1.5	1.0
Naltrexone	0.5	0.5	1.0
Diprenorphine	0.5	0.5	1.0
Antagonists "contaminated" with agonist activity			
Cyclazocine	0.9	1.5	1.7
Levallorphan	1.0	2.0	2.0
Nalorphine	1.5	4.0	2.7
Mixed agonist-antagonists			
Pentazocine	15	50	3.3
Ketocyclazocine	18	60	3.3
(−)-5-Propyl-5-nor-metazocine	12	50	4.2
(−)-5-Phenyl-5-nor-metazocine	7	30	4.3
Ethylketocyclazocine	9	59	6.4
Agonists			
Etorphine	0.5	6.0	12
Phenazocine	0.6	8.0	13
Meperidine	3000	50,000	17
Levorphanol	1.0	15	15
Methadone	7.0	200	28
Oxymorphone	1.0	30	30
Morphine	3.0	110	37
Dihydromorphine	3.0	140	47
Normorphine	15	700	47
(±)-Propoxyphene	200	12,000	60

*Relative affinity is defined by the concentration of drug required to inhibit by 50% the stereospecific binding of ^{3}H-naloxone (1.5 nM) to homogenates of rat brain minus cerebellum in the presence or absence of 100 mM NaCl. Lower affinity values indicate greater potency.
†Sodium response ratio is the ratio of the relative affinity values for inhibition by drugs of ^{3}H-naloxone binding in the presence of 100 mM NaCl to the relative affinity value in the absence of added NaCl.

exists as an equilibrium between two interconverting conformations. One conformation, which is preferred in the presence of sodium, has a greater affinity for antagonists. The other, preferred in the absence of sodium, has a greater affinity for agonists. Presumably, sodium as an

78

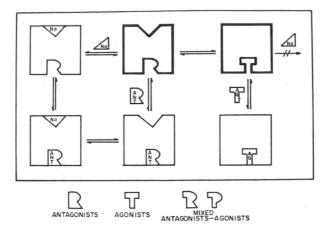

R ANTAGONISTS   T AGONISTS   R P MIXED ANTAGONISTS–AGONISTS

Figure 28. A hypothetical model of the opiate receptor based upon classic allosteric drug-receptor models. The 2 heavily outlined figures represent the 2 interconverting receptor conformations that possess differential affinities for opiate antagonists and agonists. [C. Pert]

allosteric effector drives the receptor from the agonist to the antagonist conformation (Figure 28). Thus the shift in inhibitory potency of each opiate in the presence of sodium compared to the potency in the absence of sodium is a reflection of that drug's relative affinity for the two conformations of the receptor.

Theoretical models of drug receptors in which the relative affinity for two conformational states determines intrinsic activity have been proposed (Belleau, 1964; Monod et al., 1965; Karlin, 1967; Colquhoun, 1973). Substantiation of this model in the case of the opiate receptor could be achieved only by an analysis of purified receptors. Still, Pert pointed out, a model of this type accounts for many of the perplexing pharmacological properties of opiates and provides an explanation for the "sodium effect." One can imagine how a very minor structural modification could convert an opiate that has a slightly greater affinity for the agonist conformation into one with a slightly greater affinity for the antagonist conformation, resulting in a dramatic shift in relative agonist-antagonist properties. Such a model would also account for the apparent competitive kinetics generated by opiate agonists and antagonists in vivo and in vitro, as well as the much greater potency of opiate antagonists than agonists in vivo. In the high sodium in vivo environment, the majority of the receptors would be expected to be in the "antagonist" conformation, so that relatively high concentrations of agonists would be required to drive the equilibrium in the other direction. Thus, the physiological effects of opiate agonist binding would result from the conversion of opiate receptors into an "unnatural" conformation that could no longer bind sodium. Pert wondered whether the physiological function of this opiate-sensitive, sodium-binding component is related to an ionophore, a transport mechanism, or some other, currently unimagined mechanism.

IV. NEURAL MECHANISMS

Studying the neurophysiological effects of morphine without checking their reversal by naloxone is like going to the moon and not bringing back a pebble.

F.E. Bloom

Our understanding of the neural mechanisms underlying morphine analgesia has been beset by a number of problems, in both animals and man. These problems are caused by the complexity of the pain experience as well as by the multiplicity of morphine actions. Accordingly, precise measurements are of major importance, and the presence of careful controls is essential to the correct interpretation of results. In the following sections, studies on pain and narcotics in animals and man will be discussed, followed by an examination of the structures involved in the inhibition of pain by morphine or by electrical stimulation of the brain.

Studies in Animals: F.E. Bloom

Bloom summarized several neurophysiological investigations that have been made of opiate action. Despite the appealing nature of the method, the techniques used have generally been so flawed that conclusions cannot be drawn with confidence. Many such experiments are conducted under acute surgical conditions with anesthetized animals. The use of anesthetic agents can be expected to alter the evoked response to noxious input and interact with morphine action by either potentiating or masking it.

Stereospecificity of action and reversal by antagonists are crucial tests that most investigators have omitted. Indeed, there are practically no studies in which naloxone was used to demonstrate reversibility of morphine effects on single cells in the brain. The work of Martin, demonstrating stereospecific and antagonist-reversible polysynaptic blockade by opiates in the spinal cord, is an exception (McClane and Martin, 1967a,b). Curtis and Duggan (1969) have demonstrated inhibition of cholinergic excitatory input to Renshaw cells by opiates; GABA, glycine, and glutamate effects were not blocked. The Renshaw cell, however, is not nociceptive. Dostrovsky and Pomeranz (1973) observed morphine blockade of synapses on nociceptive spinal interneurons, but the effect was nonspecific because both the inhibitory transmitters, GABA and glycine, and the excitatory transmitters, glutamate and aspartate, were affected. In these latter experiments on the spinal cord, reversibility by antagonists was not demonstrated.

Bloom's group has studied opiate actions using sucrose gap recording of the potential of dorsal and ventral root fibers of the frog spinal cord in vitro. Hyperpolarization is observed when GABA, glycine, β-alanine, or taurine is put in the bath. Morphine blocked the response to all these substances except GABA, but the effects were not stereospecific, and naloxone actually mimicked rather than antagonized the effects of morphine.

One of the few studies in which naloxone reversal was demonstrated is the work of Korf, Bunney, and Aghajanian (1974) on cells in the locus coeruleus. These cells increase in firing rate when noxious stimuli are presented, and the increase is blocked by morphine. Spontaneous activity is also inhibited. Both these effects are antagonized by naloxone. This observation gains added interest from the work of Simon on the regional distribution of the opiate receptor, which showed a high concentration of opiate binding capacity in the locus coeruleus (see above, "Opiate Receptor Binding with ^{3}H-Etorphine"). Bunney's group has found that morphine increases the spontaneous activity of neurons in the zona compacta of the substantia nigra, and this effect is also naloxone reversible. These cells, however, are not responsive to pain.*

An elegant study by Chang (1973) on the electrophysiological changes induced by morphine and acupuncture analgesia showed that after a painful stimulus both analgesic methods produce a decrease in the duration of the repetitive discharge of cells in the medial thalamus. Naloxone reversibility was not tested. On the other hand, in the spinal cord repetitive discharge of interneurons to dorsal root stimulation is blocked by morphine and appears to be restored by the antagonist levallorphan (Jurna et al., 1973). It would be most interesting if repetitive discharge in response to noxious input were blocked reversibly by morphine at several levels of the neuraxis.

*B.S. Bunney, unpublished observations.

Pain in Man: W.H. Sweet and D.J. Mayer

Although man can report verbally on his private pain experience, Mayer pointed out that we are still measuring a verbal response, not the pain itself. Response-biasing factors, such as anxiety or placebo effects, can obscure our estimation of the analgesic effects of morphine.

Matthysse stated that signal detection theory provides a novel method of analysis that is capable of correcting for response bias (Swets, 1973). Lineberry and Kulics* have applied signal detection theory to the analysis of morphine effects, and description of their experiments will indicate the essentials of the technique. Monkeys are subjected to noxious stimuli of two different strengths, and the time elapsed before an avoidance response (response latency) is recorded. For any given time interval, the probability of a response latency shorter than or equal to that interval can be computed. Actually there are two such probabilities, one for avoidance of the weaker stimulus and one for the stronger. The two probabilities are plotted (as z-scores) against each other for each time interval, one as the abscissa and the other as the ordinate. The time interval now becomes an underlying parameter but is not explicitly represented on the graph. Signal detection theory predicts that the graph should be a straight line inclined at 45°, and indeed the fit of Lineberry and Kulics's data to this prediction is remarkably good. Let us suppose that some manipulation, for example, administration of a drug, were to make the animal unable to discriminate between the stronger and weaker shocks. The line would become translated so that it passed through the origin, because the ordinate and abscissa would now be equivalent. On the other hand, suppose a manipulation were to make the animal less prompt in responding (negative response bias) without affecting his ability to discriminate. Because the time interval is only a parameter underlying the representation but does not appear on the graph, signal detection theory predicts that the new data would be represented by exactly the same straight line as before. The point corresponding to each response latency would be shifted to the left along the line, but the line itself would remain invariant. Lineberry and Kulics found that morphine did cause the line to translate toward the origin (in other words, it decreased discriminability of the two painful stimuli), and it also caused a shift along the line (negative response bias), whereas placebo caused only a shift along the line. Clark and Yang (1974) have reported that

*C.G. Lineberry and A.T. Kulics, unpublished observations.

acupuncture causes a change in response bias only, without affecting discriminability of noxious stimuli.

A major difficulty in understanding the analgesic effect of morphine on chronic pain lies in our inability to study chronic pain in the laboratory situation. Observations on chronic pain in man suggest basic differences from the acute type: (1) Thalamic lesions block chronic, but not acute, pain (Richardson and Zorub, 1970). (2) With brain stimulation, analgesia to chronic pain is longer lasting (hours) than analgesia to acute pain (about 10 min). (3) Morphine shows differential effects (more effective on chronic than on acute pain). On the other hand, the different physiological mechanisms underlying acute and chronic pain have not been elucidated.

Sweet reported that, in man, appropriately placed cerebral lesions may relieve chronic pain while sensitivity to acute pain is left intact. The sites of such lesions studied to date are predominantly limbic. That the typically intense and peculiarly intractable pain of malignant tumors may be relieved by these procedures is the best evidence we have that the relief is not just the result of suggestion or reduction of emotional tensions. Undesirable personality changes associated with large limbic lesions are avoided by making small areas of destruction. This further serves to indicate that pain relief is not simply a component of a general emotional unresponsiveness. Inferofrontal lesions have been reported by White and Sweet (1969) to produce relief in 20 of 22 cancer patients for up to 3 years, but only 3 of the patients lived more than 6 months. Other sites reported to be effective include the medial thalamus (Mark and Ervin, 1969), pulvinar (Kudo et al., 1966, 1968; Richardson and Zorub, 1970; Cooper et al., 1973), and posteromedial hypothalamus (Sano et al., 1970).

A remarkable series of 687 patients with cancer pain relieved completely in 605 instances by chemical hypophysectomy has been reported by Moricca (1974). Sweet emphasized that all these patients continue to perceive acute noxious input, while chronic pain is partially or totally relieved. However, if a new source of chronic pain emerges in such a patient, it is likely to be perceived.

Akil pointed out that such results are rather difficult to interpret because the obvious controls for lesioning, changes in anxiety or placebo effects, cannot be incorporated into the experimental design.

Aside from the methodological difficulties in measuring pain and interpretation of shifts in responsiveness, the anatomical pathways underlying pain remain obscure. It is therefore very exciting that a number of behavioral studies have yielded convergent results as to the sites of narcotic action and pain inhibition by electrical stimulation of the brain.

Anatomical Organization of Pain Pathways in the Central Nervous System: W.J.H. Nauta

Pain is classically believed to be carried along with temperature information in ascending pathways in the anterolateral funiculus of the cord. Nauta and his associates (Mehler et al., 1960) followed degenerating fibers after transection of the anterolateral quadrant of the spinal cord of the monkey in order to determine the distribution of these anterolateral fibers.

Nauta pointed out that the classical name of this tract "spinothalamic" is a *pars pro toto* term, because only a small proportion of the fibers ascend directly into the thalamus. Rather, a great many fibers appear to synapse at brainstem levels below the thalamus, largely in the tegmental reticular formation. While there is no identification of terminals in the locus coeruleus itself, the subcoeruleus nucleus, which also has a high norepinephrine content, does receive input from the anterolateral column system. A number of fibers enter the central gray midbrain substance; this connection was orignially reported by Clark (1932) as the spino-annular tract. Nauta recalled Bechterew's (1900) view that the central gray substance can be seen as a "nodal point" in conduction pathways, and as such may constitute the lowest level at which pain is integrated. Pathways from the central gray ascend to the hypothalamus and connect this area with the limbic system, possibly playing an important role in integrating the emotional characteristics of pain.

The small number of truly "spinothalamic" fibers of this system terminate in two different regions of the thalamus:

1. Terminations in the ventral basal region of the thalamus: In monkey and man, spinothalamic fibers terminate in a remarkably spotty ("archipelago") fashion within the nucleus ventralis posterolateralis (VPL). This tract overlays to a certain extent the terminations of the medial lemniscus, a parallel ascending system conveying tactile and proprioceptive information. This region therefore represents an area of convergence between the medial lemniscus and the spinothalamic tract and represents the thalamic gateway to the somatosensory

cortex. It is possible that this "neospinothalamic" component of the pathway contributes the quality of sharpness to pain.

2. Terminations in the intralaminar nuclei of the thalamus: Other fibers of the anterolateral funiculus of the cord terminate in the nonspecific nuclei paracentralis and centralis lateralis of the thalamus, in what appear to be small clusters of cells. Part of these fibers decussate in the posterior commissure and terminate in the contralateral intralaminar nuclei. These medial spinothalamic fibers may be homologous to the spino-diencephalic system of lower vertebrates and have been referred to as the *paleo*spinothalamic tract.

The exact projections of these pathways past the thalamus remain vague. Projections from the intralaminar nuclei terminate diffusely in the cortex; their afferent connections are highly diverse and include, besides spinothalamic fibers, projections from the cerebellum and from large regions of the reticular brainstem tegmentum.

The terminations in the specific nuclei of the ventrobasal complex of the thalamus may not represent the major aspects of pain that Medicine tries to deal with: ablation of the somatic sensory cortex, the apparent ultimate target of this conduction system, has long been known to be ineffective in attempts to relieve pain. Although this connection may subserve the spatial coding of the specific sensory component of "fast pain," it probably is not (or only in lesser degree) involved in the "suffering" produced by chronic pain, a state that interferes with sleep, pleasure, autonomic functioning, ideation, and the ability of an organism to attend to other perceptions. Such pain constitutes a change in the whole internal set of the organism, an existential state rather than a sensory one. While morphine may not block the epicritic elements of acute pain, it appears to reduce this "suffering," possibly by blocking an outflow from the nociceptive pathway to the limbic structures.

Discussion centered around explaining the role of the central gray and intralaminar nuclei in mediating the pain inhibition produced by microinjections of morphine or electrical stimulation in these areas.

When asked if he regarded the central gray core from the periaqueductal to the periventricular and medial thalamic area as a functional unit, Nauta replied that, although a definitive answer to this question would have to await further physiological studies, such a unison is indeed suggested by the reciprocal connections established between the central gray substance of the midbrain and the periventricular region of the diencephalon by the dorsal longitudinal fasciculus of Schütz. Another connection of possible importance in the pain mechanism consists of the fibers of Weisschedel's "radiatio grisca tegmenti" (Nauta, 1958), which connect the central gray substance with a very large cross-sectional area of the midbrain tegmentum: It could be that this radiation connects in part with pathways descending to the medulla and spinal cord that affect the transmission of nociceptive impulses at an early stage of synaptic processing. A. Pert pointed out that there are also ascending connections from central gray to the intralaminar nuclei, which may constitute a further ascending influence through which pain inhibition is achieved by central gray stimulation (Figure 29).

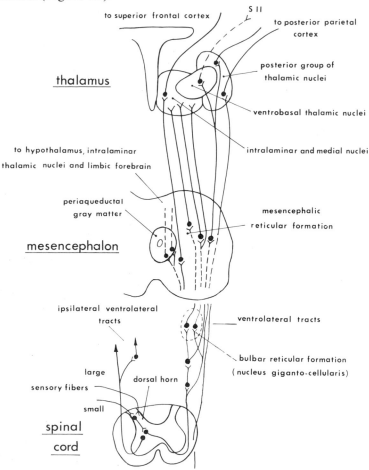

Figure 29. The extralemniscal somatosensory pathways. [Adapted by A. Pert from Melzack, 1973]

Since this Work Session took place, new anatomical evidence has been published that may contribute to a better understanding of the functional role of the periaqueductal-periventricular system in pain and analgesia.

Histofluorescence work, employing the more sensitive glyoxylic acid technique, has demonstrated that the ascending portion of the dorsal longitudinal fasciculus of Schütz is rich in catecholamines (Lindvall et al., 1974). This catecholaminergic system, termed the dorsal periventricular bundle, appears to arise in the raphe region and the central gray area of the mesencephalon, innervates the midline thalamic and hypothalamic areas, and terminates in the thalamic, epithalamic, and pretectal regions.

Both A. Pert's microinjection and Mayer's stimulation studies (see below) point to the importance of the periaqueductal-periventricular system in analgesia. The fact that these areas involve a well-integrated catecholamine system may help focus our efforts in studying the role of dopamine and norepinephrine in the modulation of pain.

Analgesia Produced by Morphine Microinjections in the Primate Brain: A. Pert

A number of studies employing microinjection techniques have underlined the importance of certain brain areas in mediating opiate analgesia. Studies by Tsou and Jang (1964) in the rabbit and by Jacquet and Lajtha (1973) in the rat have pointed to the area surrounding the third ventricle as a primary site of action of morphine. Buxbaum and his co-workers (1970) implicate the anterior thalamus, while Herz and his collaborators (1970) believe that structures in the floor of the fourth ventricle are the primary loci of action of morphine. Thus, in rodents, the analgesic sites appear to be medially located within periventricular and periaqueductal structures in the brainstem and diencephalon. Pert examined the sites of morphine action in the monkey and compared them with the localization of opiate receptor binding sites and the anatomical pathways involved in the processing of pain.

In Pert's studies, rhesus monkeys are implanted with 4 to 6 bilateral pairs of 22 ga microinjection guides. Brain sites are mapped for antinociceptive activity by injections of 1.0 or 2.0 μl of a solution containing 20 µg of morphine. Injections are made through 27 ga injectors at successively greater depths past the tip of the guide in increments of 2 or 3 mm. Up to 50 sites can be mapped in a single animal with this technique. Analgesia is measured by the shock titration technique of Weiss and Laties (1970). Briefly, electrical shock to the feet of restrained monkeys is increased progressively every 2 seconds in fixed increments. Each lever press by the animal reduces the shock by the same amount. The analgesic threshold is defined as that shock level beneath which the animal spends 90% of its time. This level corresponds well with the escape threshold in the same animal.

Under control conditions, the animal usually keeps the shock level at 0.5 mA. After an injection of 20 µg of morphine into a morphine-responsive site, the shock threshold shows a gradual increase that reaches an asymptotic level in 3 to 4 hours. Naloxone was found to reverse these effects of morphine immediately when injected intravenously in a dose of 1 to 5 mg/kg. By contrast, 20 µg of dextrorphan injected into the identical site produces no effect. Interestingly, etorphine in a 1 µg dose produces an immediate and potent analgesic effect that subsides in 15 min. The rapid effect of etorphine is probably due to the fact that it is 300 times more lipid soluble than morphine. Similarly, the slow onset of action of morphine derives from the requirement of this opiate, which is not very lipid soluble, to diffuse over a critical mass of brain tissue. This critical mass appears to be about 3 mm in diameter, measured as a sphere.

Results obtained by these microinjection experiments are not due to diffusion of the drug into the ventricle, because no more than 10% of the morphine injected into the periaqueductal gray reaches the ventricle. Direct application of this amount into the ventricle does not produce analgesia.

The specificity of localization is further indicated in Figure 30, which shows that more dorsal sites in the thalamus do not cause analgesia, whereas the periventricular injection brings about a long-lasting effect, reversible by naloxone.

Using these techniques, Pert and Yaksh (1974a,b, 1975) have mapped over 500 sites in the rhesus monkey brain. The region of the brain that is most enriched in analgesic sites is the periventricular-periaqueductal gray matter (lateral ventricles 1.0 and 2.0 of Figure 31). It extends from the lower portion of the third ventricle along the aqueduct into the fourth ventricle. Several sites, also located near the midline, are seen along the ventrolateral borders of the centromedian and parafascicular nuclei of the thalamus. A second morphine-sensitive

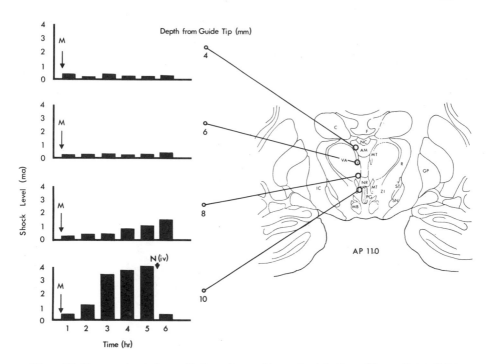

Figure 30. Neuroanatomical specificity of morphine microinjection. 20 μg of morphine injected at 4 different depths from the tip of the guide cannula at AP plane 11.0. For a definition of abbreviations, see Figure 31. [A. Pert]

brain region occurs in a more lateral area about 5 mm from midline in an area ranging from the substantia nigra, through the red nucleus, up to the intralaminar region of the thalamus. Some of these sites are as caudal as the pons. These more lateral sites are not as active as the medial ones (Figure 31).

Pert indicated that there is a positive correlation between the effective analgesic sites in the brain and those areas found to be rich in opiate receptor binding sites by Kuhar and co-workers (1973) and by Hiller and his colleagues (1973). Thus, the areas of the medial thalamus, periaqueductal and periventricular gray matter, and hypothalamus that are rich in opiate receptor binding sites appear to be most effective in producing analgesia when injected with morphine. The major discrepancy appears to be in the amygdala, an area rich in opiate binding in which morphine was found to be ineffective.

Pert noted that the amygdala may mediate more subtle aspects of pain appreciation or that it may mediate other effects of opiates. Nauta concurred that opiate receptors in the amygdala might not be related to the analgesic properties but to other pharmacological actions

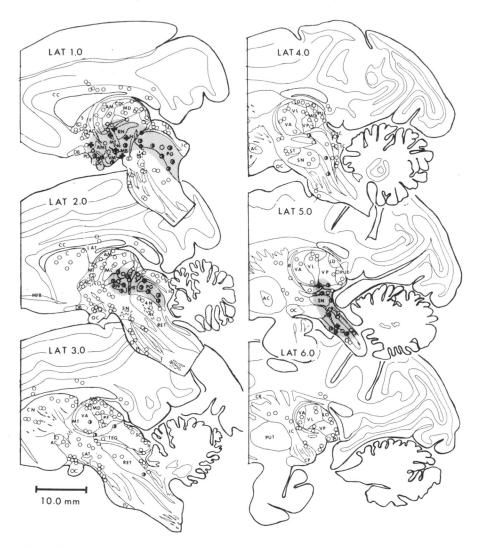

Figure 31. Anatomical mapping of the analgesic sites of action of morphine in the primate brain at 6 sagittal levels from the midline in 1 mm increments (LAT 1.0 to LAT 6.0). ○ = no response following 40 μg injection; ⊙ = sites that produced a threshold increase of greater than 0.64 mA but less than 1.6; + = maximally active sites in which injections of the mapping dose resulted in a threshold shift of 1.6 mA or more. The active regions have been shaded in gray. AC = anterior commissure; AM = nucleus anterior medialis; ANT = anterior hypothalamic area; CC = corpus callosum; CDC = nucleus centralis densocellularis; CM = nucleus centrum medianum; CN = caudate nucleus; CP = cerebral peduncle; DB = diagonal band of Broca; F = fornix; GP = globus pallidus; HI = hippocampus; IC = internal capsule; LAT = lateral ventricle; LD = nucleus lateralis dorsalis; MB = mammillary body; MD = nucleus medialis dorsalis; MFB = medial forebrain bundle; MT = mammillo-thalamic tract; OC = optic chiasm; PF = nucleus parafascicularis; PG = periaqueductal gray matter; PO = preoptic area; PUL = pulvinar thalami; PUT = putamen; R = nucleus reticularis; RET = reticular formation; RN = nucleus reuniens; S = septum pellucidium; SC = superior colliculus; SN = substantia nigra; ST = subthalamic nucleus; TEG = tegmentum; VA = nucleus ventralis anterior; VL = nucleus ventralis lateralis; VM = ventromedial nucleus; VP = nucleus ventralis posterior. [Pert and Yaksh, 1974b]

of morphine such as tranquility and passive euphoria, somewhat reminiscent of the placidity that has been observed in cats and monkeys following certain lesions of the amygdala.

Pert went on to emphasize that the loci of his active sites also correlated well with structures served by pain pathways arising from the anterolateral columns of the spinal cord as described by Nauta and reported by Mehler, Feferman, and Nauta (1960). The central gray area is a relay point from the extralemniscal system to the limbic area and may act as a switch mechanism interfacing the sensory and emotional aspects of pain. The other effective area is the medial thalamus and intralaminar nuclei around the third ventricle. This corresponds to the nonspecific projection area of the spinothalamic tract, the system termed "paleospinothalamic" by Nauta. This phylogenetically older system is slower, polysynaptic, with long-lasting afterdischarge, and is thought to underlie the protopathic aspects of pain. It is these aspects that are blocked by morphine. The more acute, epicritic pain aspects are processed by the part of the spinothalamic pathway that projects to the ventrobasal complex and is termed "neospinothalamic." Here again, the correlation is good, because morphine does not usually block the epicritic aspects of pain, and injections of morphine in the ventrobasal complex of the thalamus fail to elicit analgesia.

Furthermore, these periaqueductal and periventricular areas have been implicated in the appreciation of pain by a number of other findings. Acute electrical stimulation of the periaqueductal gray region (Olds and Olds, 1963; Skultety, 1963) and the medial and intralaminar thalamic nuclei (Kaelber and Mitchell, 1967) has produced aversive reactions indicative of pain in a number of species, including man (Nashold et al., 1969). Lesions in the central gray region and the intralaminar thalamic nuclei, on the other hand, have resulted in moderate analgesia (Melzack et al., 1958; Mitchell and Kaelber, 1966; Anderson and Mahan, 1971). More recent studies (Mayer et al., 1971; Liebeskind et al., 1973) have reported analgesia from prolonged stimulation of the periventricular-periaqueductal gray matter. In Pert's work, stimulation of morphine-sensitive sites with electrodes introduced through the guide cannulae was ineffective in producing analgesia.

Morphine microinjection appears to be a useful tool in investigating the neuroanatomical loci of narcotic action. The effective sites seem to correlate well with the distribution of opiate binding sites in the brain as well as with areas served by the paleospinothalamic and spinoreticular fibers of the extralemniscal system.

Neuroanatomical Correlates of Morphine Dependence:
A. Herz

A number of different sites of action have to be considered for the acute effects of opiates. One might suggest that all these morphine-sensitive structures develop tolerance and dependence. Thus it would follow that all these sites contribute to the morphine withdrawal symptomatology. Until now only a few investigations have dealt with the neuroanatomical correlates of morphine dependence. Studies of lesions of distinct brain areas are of limited value in determining the primary site of morphine action because the effects on secondarily involved centers or pathways cannot be differentiated. The evaluation of sites of action of opiate antagonists precipitating withdrawal, however, can lead to conclusions concerning the primary site of action of morphine itself.

It has been shown (Herz et al., 1972) that in morphine-dependent rabbits, severe withdrawal signs are precipitated when morphine antagonists are administered into the fourth ventricle. However, the withdrawal symptomatology is rather weak because the antagonists can spread only in the anterior portions of the ventricular system. Recently Wei and his colleagues (1973a) obtained results in rats pointing to mesodiencephalic sites of action of naloxone in the precipitation of withdrawal. In recent investigations, Herz's group also used rats to quantitate a series of withdrawal signs (Laschka et al., 1974). In comparing the withdrawal pattern precipitated by intraventricular administration of opiate antagonists with the pattern of signs precipitated by systemic administration, only minor qualitative differences can be observed. (Writhing and diarrhea are the only signs not well developed with intraventricular administration.) However, the antagonist was found to be effective at much lower doses when applied directly into the ventricular system than when given systemically. From this result, Herz concludes that most withdrawal signs originate from brain sites easily reached from the ventricular space.

To define the periventricular site of action more accurately, the antagonists were applied to restricted parts of the ventricular system, adapting a method developed for the rabbit (Albus, 1972). It was found that injections of naloxone (or levallorphan) into the fourth ventricle are much more effective in eliciting abstinence signs than injections into the lateral and third ventricle, provided the drug is prevented by a plug from diffusing into the lower parts of the ventricular system (Fig-

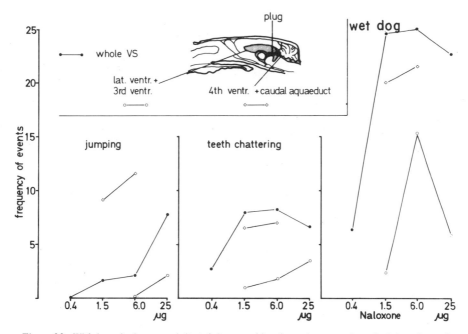

Figure 32. Withdrawal signs precipitated in morphine-dependent rats by administration of naloxone into restricted parts of the ventricular system (VS). The rats were subcutaneously implanted with 6 morphine pellets (75 mg morphine) within 10 days. A eucerine plug was inserted into the aqueductus mesencephali. When naloxone was injected into the lateral ventricle, it could spread in both lateral ventricles and the third ventricle; when injected into the fourth ventricle, it could also reach the lower parts of the aqueduct. For comparison, data obtained by naloxone injection into the unplugged ventricular system are also given. [Laschka]

ure 32). The anterior part of the floor of the fourth ventricle and caudal region of the periaqueductal gray matter are most critical as sites of action of the antagonists; this is especially true for jumping, an important withdrawal sign. Whether signs such as wet dog shaking also originate in structures lining the anterior parts of the ventricular system cannot be decided from these experiments. In any case, structures easily reached from the fourth ventricle seem to be more sensitive in eliciting this sign. Microinjection of levallorphan into the caudate nucleus is ineffective in producing withdrawal signs in morphine-dependent rats; when levallorphan is injected into the medial areas of the thalamus, weak withdrawal signs are precipitated. Experiments with tritium-labeled levallorphan injected into medial thalamic regions show the presence of radioactivity in the cerebrospinal fluid in those experiments in which more than very weak withdrawal signs can be observed. Accordingly, one must be exceedingly cautious with the microinjection technique in order to rule out migration of the drug from the brain tissue through the cerebrospinal fluid to other sites of the brain.

A. Pert also feels that one cannot map withdrawal sites in the brain with the highly lipid-soluble opiate antagonists such as naloxone. He found that radioactive naloxone diffuses extremely rapidly throughout brain tissue. Within 15 min after a microinjection of ^{3}H-naloxone, negligible amounts remain at the site of injection.

Pain Inhibition by Electrical Brain Stimulation: Comparison to Morphine: D.J. Mayer

Mayer chose to focus on three issues. The first involved a description of analgesia induced by electrical stimulation. Secondly, he described a number of studies in which he compared this phenomenon to morphine analgesia, suggesting commonalities in the underlying mechanisms. Finally, he advanced a simple model to summarize the various findings.

Stimulation-Induced Analgesia

Electrical stimulation of certain areas in the brain can produce very powerful analgesia in rats and cats (Mayer et al., 1971; Liebeskind et al., 1973). When stimulated in the effective areas, animals become totally unresponsive to pain while retaining a normal ability to respond to other stimuli. Numerous experiments have been conducted to rule out other possible explanations. This analgesia is not due to a functional lesion at the stimulation site, since actual electrolytic lesions produce very different effects. Neither is it due to the production of focal seizures, since recordings from these areas immediately after stimulation do not reveal such activity (Mayer and Liebeskind, 1974). There is no overall decrease in motor responsiveness, and other reflexes of the animal remain intact. In fact, brain stimulation can produce analgesia in certain parts of the body, leaving responsiveness in other areas quite intact (Mayer et al., 1971). Moreover, the analgesic sites are not necessarily correlated with areas that are positively reinforcing to the animal. Such behavioral observations indicate that the lack of response to pain is quite specific and cannot be attributed to lesioning, seizure, distraction, or generalized lack of responsiveness. Interestingly, the analgesic effect outlasts brain stimulation from a few minutes to several hours, depending on the duration and intensity of stimulation.

This technique of pain blockade has recently been used clinically in patients suffering from intractable pain as a nondestructive alternative to the lesioning procedures usually employed (Richardson and Akil, 1974).

Parallels to Narcotic Analgesia

A fascinating aspect of stimulation-induced analgesia is its similarity to certain aspects of morphine analgesic action. Both are thought to involve an active process of pain inhibition, rather than merely the blockade of pain input. For example, narcotics appear to be dependent on the integrity of brain neurotransmitters for their action (Way and Shen, 1971). There is evidence that stimulation-produced analgesia is also modulated by monoaminergic transmission (Akil et al., 1972). It appears to be facilitated by serotonin, particularly in those sites close to the dorsal raphe (Akil and Mayer, 1972); it is further facilitated by dopamine and antagonized by norepinephrine.

The most striking parallel between stimulation analgesia and morphine analgesia lies in their sites of action. As A. Pert has indicated, the best analgesic loci for morphine microinjections lie along the periaqueductal and periventricular gray areas. Similarly, stimulation analgesia is most readily obtained from sites extending from the fourth ventricle along the aqueduct and around the third ventricle, including the intralaminar nuclei of the thalamus. It is on the basis of such evidence that Mayer and Liebeskind (1974) have theorized that both morphine and brain stimulation activate a common pain inhibitory mechanism in the brain, a mechanism that may also be modulated by other analgesic techniques, by emotional and motivational changes, and by hypnosis. This theory predicts that brain stimulation analgesia should show further similarities to narcotics such as blockade by narcotic antagonists and development of tolerance.

Akil, Mayer, and Liebeskind (1972) have performed several experiments to determine the effects of naloxone on stimulation analgesia. The tail-flick method was used to measure baseline pain responses and changes induced by pain stimulation. Tail-flick testing occurred immediately upon termination of the stimulation. On the control day, animals were preinjected with saline; brain stimulation was administered that rendered each animal totally analgesic by an operationally defined criterion. Two days later, the animals were injected with naloxone (1 mg/kg) and tested in a similar fashion.

96

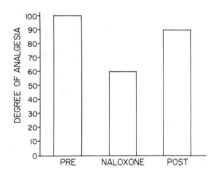

Figure 33. Effect of naloxone on stimulation-produced analgesia. Pretest gives degree of analgesia present with control injection of saline. Naloxone (1 mg/kg) was given 2 days later, 0.5 h before testing. Another saline control was run 2 days after naloxone (post-test). [Mayer]

Finally, they were retested two days after naloxone with saline injection (Figure 33). Naloxone produced a significant antagonism of analgesia, reducing it from 100% to 60%. Analgesia returned to 90% two days after naloxone treatment.

This naloxone effect has been obtained repeatedly and with lower analgesic levels. However, there appears to be a limit to the reversal, since an increase in naloxone dose does not produce total reversal.

Stimulation-produced analgesia is also subject to tolerance. After continuous stimulation for 24 hours, there is a significant decrease in the analgesic effectiveness of stimulation. Upon termination of stimulation, the analgesic effect recovers gradually over 2 weeks. This "tolerance" is never complete, analgesia usually being reduced between 30% and 60% of its initial level.

Continuous stimulation is not necessary for the production of tolerance. Daily stimulation lasting 60 seconds leads to tolerance that appears on the second day and reaches a maximum level after 5 to 7 days.

There is also some evidence of cross-tolerance. Analgesic brain stimulation loses its effectiveness in blocking pain if the animal is made tolerant to narcotics by daily systemic injections of morphine. On the other hand, tolerance to brain stimulation does not prevent subsequent analgesia by morphine injection. This is not surprising, since morphine acts at all analgesia-producing sites in the brain, whereas electrical stimulation affects only one. Thus, brain stimulation shares many of the properties of morphine action, exhibiting blockade by narcotic antagonists, tolerance, and cross-tolerance with morphine.

Schematic Model of Pain Inhibition

Figure 34 shows a schematic model that Mayer introduced to account for these results. To begin with, there is a pain input at the spinal level that eventually ascends along pathways described above by Nauta. This input projects, in a somatotopic fashion, into the central gray matter with the tail being represented maximally, followed by the hind limbs, then the forelimbs (Liebeskind and Mayer, 1971). Noxious input is inhibited by central gray stimulation following the same somatotopic pattern (Mayer and Liebeskind, 1974).

A portion of the pain inhibitory systems appears to be ascending, because it involves the dopaminergic system known to ascend into the brain without descending into the cord. The descending part into the cord may involve serotonin as the inhibitory transmitter, since this substance appears important for analgesia and has a segmental

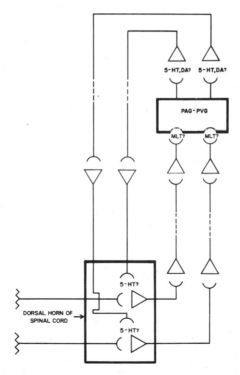

Figure 34. Theoretical model of neural circuitry and neurohumoral substances involved in stimulation-produced analgesia. PAG = periaqueductal gray matter; PVG = periventricular gray matter; MLT = morphine-like transmitter; DA = dopamine. [Mayer]

distribution in the cord paralleling the somatotopy of pain input and inhibition, with 5-hydroxytryptamine terminals concentrated mostly in the sacral regions and least in the cervical segments.

The most speculative aspect of the model is the "morphine-like" transmitter around the periaqueductal-periventricular areas. The presence of such a substance was proposed by Hughes and others in this meeting. If such a substance exists, it would be released by electrical stimulation in the gray core of the brain. It would be expected that this released material would be antagonized by naloxone, and that the system may be subject to tolerance, as reported by Mayer. The fact that neither the naloxone blockade nor the tolerance effects are complete may be due to stimulation of some elements located postsynaptically to the terminals releasing a "morphine-like" substance, thus directly activating the pain inhibitory system. This direct activation would not be blocked by antagonists.

Acupuncture may act in a similar fashion, Mayer speculated, by eventually releasing this same substance in the brain and leading to pain inhibition. In this case, however, the activation would be entirely presynaptic, and naloxone would produce a total reversal of this analgesic effect.

Mayer also reported preliminary experiments done in collaboration with Donald Price, indicating that acupuncture analgesia in humans is reversible by naloxone (Figure 35). Five minutes after naloxone

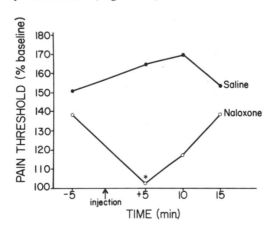

Figure 35. Effect of naloxone on acupuncture analgesia. Pain threshold is represented as % baseline pain threshold for tooth pulp stimulation. Thresholds are given 5 min before and 5, 10, and 15 min after either saline or 0.8 mg naloxone administered intravenously. * indicates a significant difference between pre-injection analgesia and post-injection analgesia (p = .005; one-tailed t-test). Six subjects were in naloxone group and 4 in the saline group. [Mayer]

administration, analgesia obtained from stimulation of the Hoku point*
was abolished, whereas in the saline control group the effect persisted.
The naloxone blockade lasted 15 min. However, the interpretation of
these observations is still uncertain.

Discussion of Neural Mechanisms of Analgesia

The convergence of information concerning the critical sites for
analgesia appears striking. Results of widely different techniques such
as opiate binding, morphine microinjections, and electrical stimulation
all indicate the importance of the mesencephalic central gray area and
sites surrounding the third and fourth ventricle, particularly the area of
the nonspecific nuclei of the thalamus. Anatomically these regions are
known to receive input from the pathways carrying pain and
temperature information and appear crucial in the processing of
protopathic pain and its emotional components.

What may be unclear, however, is exactly how pain inhibition
occurs along these sites. As A. Pert indicated, lesioning of these areas
can produce pain relief. Mayer has reported that stimulation of these
sites is analgesic, whereas others have found stimulation in these areas
to be noxious. These apparent contradictions are resolved if the
stimulation parameters are specified. In the human, electrical stimulation of the intralaminar nuclei is analgesic if it remains at low
frequencies (10 to 20 Hz) and low amplitude (Richardson and Akil,
1974); increasing the frequency or the amplitude leads to noxious
effects. The patients never report specific pain; rather they describe
arousal, anxiety, and a need to escape. Whatever pain relief may still
exist is totally masked by these emotions. On the other hand, low-level
stimulation produces a feeling of relaxation and well-being. It seems
obvious from these observations that the functions of these areas are
mixed. Whatever mechanism inhibits pain appears to run closely with
the pain pathway but exhibits a different stimulation threshold. Pain
may be inhibited by actually transecting or lesioning the sensory
pathways, or it may be blocked by activating the low-threshold
inhibitory mechanism built into the system. It is worth noting that this
same interaction exists at the periphery, whereby low-intensity peripheral nerve stimulation activates the larger fibers and produces analgesia;

*The Hoku point is located between the thumb and index finger at the approximate center of
the interosseus dorsalis I muscle.

increasing the frequency and amplitude activates the small fibers and produces pain.

The above observations suggest that pain must proceed along the nervous system under the control of facilitatory and inhibitory influences. Presumably, core gray regions would be the starting point for pain inhibitory loops that may be short and regional, altering pain processing at their own level of the neuraxis, or long and more complex, including ascending systems that modulate the interpretation of the emotional-perceptual characteristics of pain, and descending influences that close the sensory "gate" and alter input at the first synapse.

The fact that these areas of integration are rich in narcotic binding sites may be very significant. It is tempting to speculate, along with Hughes and others at this meeting, that a naturally occurring substance exists in the same sites where opiate binding is found. It is unclear whether morphine would activate the receptor in a fashion agonistic or antagonistic to this endogenous substance. It may be noted, however, that in Hughes's experiments on the vas deferens, the extract of the endogenous substance affected the preparation in a morphine-like fashion. It is therefore possible that low-frequency brain stimulation releases this substance, whereas morphine mimics its effect on the receptor. Obviously, these speculations could be tested once an endogenous substance has been identified and its interactions with morphine examined. At that point, the judicious use of electrical stimulation and microinjection techniques in combination may be invaluable in pinpointing secondary sites and mechanisms essential in the production of analgesia tolerance and dependence. It is likely that our difficulties in understanding pain are partially due to our lack of understanding of its inhibitory mechanisms. The recent experimental and theoretical advances in the field of narcotics may constitute the first step towards answering the puzzle of pain.

V. BIOCHEMICAL PHENOMENA
IN OPIATE ACTION AND ADDICTION

Goldstein and Bloom addressed themselves to the unknown biochemical events that mediate between the combination of an opiate with its receptor and the occurrence of opiate-specific behavioral effects. These as yet undetermined mechanisms were subsumed under the term "the black box" by Goldstein and Bloom (Figure 36). They pointed out that many biochemical alterations occur during opiate administration, but it is unclear whether any of these changes are related in a causal way to the production of analgesia or the processes of tolerance and physical dependence. A number of approaches to this problem have been attempted:

1. Determination of biochemical alterations occurring directly at the cellular level following opiate administration. Such studies in the past have noted changes in the brain levels or turnover of neurotransmitter substances, formation of cyclic adenosine monophosphate (cAMP), changes in the energy metabolism, phospholipid, protein, or nucleic acid metabolism (for review see Clouet, 1971a). However, when considering any biochemical approach, a change occurring in a system concurrent with the administration of an opiate should be considered opiate specific only if it is antagonized by treatment with naloxone, is shown to be stereospecific, and occurs with a reasonably low concentration of the opiate. These criteria have often not been met, and many contradictory conclusions have been drawn.

2. Pharmacological manipulations of the guinea pig ileum or mouse vas deferens in vitro models to modify the action of opiates on these preparations.

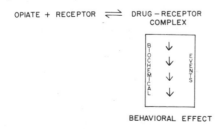

Figure 36. Sequence of events following opiate-receptor combination. The opiate ligand is thought to alter receptor conformation, thus leading to modification of an unknown biochemical pathway, the end result of which is the observed behavioral effect. For example, the opiate-receptor combination could result in inhibition of a specific adenylate cyclase. [Goldstein]

3. Pharmacological manipulation of in vivo biochemical systems with observations of changes in the behavioral response of animals after acute opiate administration, during development of tolerance and dependence, and modification of withdrawal symptoms precipitated by naloxone.

Biochemical Processes in Addiction: H.H. Loh

Loh studied the mechanisms related to changes in protein synthesis occurring during morphine administration. Clouet (1971b) had described an increase in protein synthesis that correlated with the addictive process; however, her studies involved total protein synthesis. Loh examined specific macromolecules that might be related in a selective fashion to the process of tolerance and physical dependence. Chronic morphine treatment increases the template activity of mouse brain chromatin. In tolerant mice, 3 days after morphine pellet implantation there is almost twice as much incorporation of radioactive uridine triphosphate (UTP) into DNA as compared to nontolerant animals (Figure 37). Animals pretreated with naloxone prior to the implantation of morphine pellets do not show any increase in chromatin template activity. This fulfills one of the criteria of an opiate-specific effect. However, the specificity of this effect was questioned by Matthysse and C. Pert, who suggested that Loh should determine whether a variety of drugs unrelated to opiates, such as amphetamine or barbiturates, might also increase chromatin template

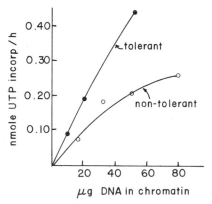

Figure 37. The rate of UTP incorporation with various amounts of chromatin isolated from tolerant or nontolerant mice. The rate of UTP incorporation is expressed as nmole/h. [Loh]

activity via secondary effects caused by changes, for example, in locomotor activity.

To evaluate the mechanism of the increase in template activity, Loh removed the histones from the chromatin. This did not alter the results of the investigation. In fact, the electrophoretic pattern of the histones was not altered in opiate-addicted animals. Salt extraction was used to remove selectively the acidic proteins, and electrophoresis demonstrated the presence of a unique acidic nonhistone protein that was synthesized in the brains of addicted mice.

Way emphasized the role that protein synthesis may play in the development of tolerance and dependence. Administration of cycloheximide, a protein synthesis inhibitor, will block the development of tolerance to and physical dependence on morphine, at a dose that does not modify the antinociceptive response to morphine (Loh et al., 1969) (Figure 38). He interpreted this result to mean that the protein or macromolecule concerned with tolerance and dependence development is not the morphine receptor at the effector site but some other protein with a more rapid rate of turnover. Of course, one must be cautious about ascribing an effect of cycloheximide to inhibition of protein synthesis, because this drug has myriad other actions.

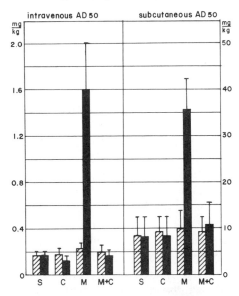

Figure 38. Cycloheximide inhibition of morphine tolerance development. Tolerance is evidenced by the increase in the dose (AD_{50}) of morphine (M) required to produce analgesia after its repeated administration for several days. Cycloheximide (C) and saline (S) were also injected daily. [Loh et al., 1969]

Effects of Drugs on Neurotransmitter Systems:
A.J. Mandell

Mandell addressed himself to the biochemical changes that occur during acute morphine administration in central nervous system (CNS) neurotransmitter systems. There is a massive literature on attempts to connect the pharmacological effects of opiates with the biogenic amines in the brain (for review see Clouet, 1971a). In the past, attention had been focused on changes occurring in the whole-brain content of norepinephrine, dopamine, or serotonin, and therefore the data had been inconclusive as to the precise role that these transmitter systems play in the mediation of opiate effects. Much research has indicated that changes in the dynamic mechanisms in the rate of synthesis or reuptake of neurotransmitters may have a greater relevance to drug effects than the steady-state levels of these substances, and that such changes may be different in various brain regions.

Mandell has been studying drug effects on brain neurotransmitter systems through the use of multiple measures that include (1) soluble enzyme activity in cell bodies, (2) high-affinity uptake of precursor in nerve endings, (3) soluble enzyme activity after lysis in nerve endings, and (4) synaptosomal conversion of precursors to neurotransmitter substances. He restricted his discussion to changes in the serotonin system, which has cell bodies in the raphe nuclei and innervates the septum and corpus striatum (Knapp and Mandell, 1972). Morphine increases synaptosomal conversion of tryptophan to serotonin 90 min after administration (Figure 39). This increase is not caused by an alteration in tryptophan uptake. Surprisingly, the activity of tryptophan hydroxylase in the lysed synaptosomal preparation is decreased by 60%. Naloxone at an equivalent dose has no effect, while nalorphine produces inconsistent changes in this preparation, which may reflect its partial agonist properties. In contrast to morphine, amphetamine and reserpine do not produce morphine-like effects on serotonin formation. Whereas amphetamine also elicits an immediate decrease in synaptosomal tryptophan hydroxylase activity, this is accompanied by an equivalent decrease in the conversion of tryptophan to serotonin. These results emphasize the necessity of multiple measures of drug-induced changes in transmitter systems before meaningful comparisons of mechanisms of action can be made.

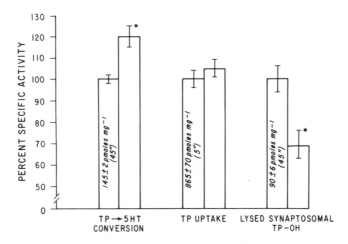

Figure 39. The effects of morphine sulfate (15 mg/kg, 90 min before sacrifice) on measures of serotonin synthesis in rat striatum, expressed as % of control specific activity (left column in each pair). *, experimental values that were significantly different from their respective control values. TP-5HT conversion refers to synaptosomal conversion of ^{14}C-tryptophan to $^{14}CO_2$ plus serotonin (determined stoichiometrically). TP uptake refers to synaptosomal retention of L-3-^{14}C-tryptophan (10 μM) after incubation at 37°C for 4 min. Lysed synaptosomal TP-OH refers to the activity of tryptophan hydroxylase solubilized from striate synaptosomes. [Mandell]

Interactions Between Opiates and Other Neuroactive Substances: Prostaglandins and Serotonin: J.M. Musacchio

Musacchio reviewed his results on the failure of prostaglandins (PG) to participate in the inhibitory response to morphine of the guinea pig ileum in vitro model. Ehrenpreis and his collaborators (1973) had claimed that PGE_1 and PGE_2 were essential for the release of acetylcholine in the guinea pig ileum. This assumption was based on the observation that indomethacin, a potent PG-synthesis inhibitor, blocked the response of the guinea pig ileum to electrical stimulation; this inhibition was reversed only by the addition of PGE_1 or PGE_2. The inhibitory effects of morphine on the gut were believed by Ehrenpreis and his colleagues to derive from the narcotic's ability to compete for the PG receptor and thereby prevent release of acetylcholine. However, the results in Musacchio's laboratory are at complete variance with previous work.* Musacchio showed that PGE_2 by itself causes a

*A.R. Gintzler and J.M. Musacchio, unpublished observation.

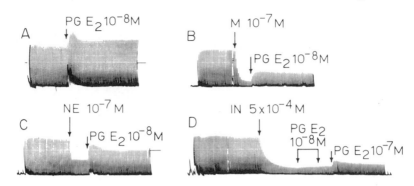

Figure 40. Effects of PGE_2 on the inhibitory response to morphine (M), norepinephrine (NE), and indomethacin (IN). Effects of PGE_2 on the response of the guinea pig ileum to electrical stimulation (A), morphine sulfate (B), norepinephrine (C), and indomethacin (D). All the drugs were added directly into the 50 ml organ bath such that the final molarity was as indicated. In D the content of PGE_2 is cumulative since there was no washing between the 3 additions of PGE_2. After the effect of each drug was determined, the preparation was washed 3 times at 1 min intervals and allowed to rest for 12 min before the next addition was made. [Gintzler and Musacchio]

sustained increase in the response to electrical stimulation (Figure 40A). Although PGE_2 can partially reverse the inhibition produced by morphine, it is even more effective in partially reversing the inhibition produced by a similar concentration of norepinephrine (Figure 40B and C). Since PGE_2 alone can cause an increase in the response to electrical stimulation, and since it can also partially antagonize the inhibitory effects of morphine and norepinephrine, it appears likely that any antagonism by PGE_2 might be nonspecific.

Indomethacin does cause a pronounced inhibition of the response to electrical stimulation (Figure 40D). However this inhibition is not reversed by PGE_2 at a concentration as high as 1×10^{-7} M. This would imply that the inhibition produced by indomethacin is independent of its effects on the synthesis of prostaglandins and cannot be used as evidence to support a postulated endogenous function for PGE_1 or PGE_2.

A more direct way to dissociate the inhibitory effects of indomethacin from its effects on synthesis of PG is to assay the activity of prostaglandin dioxygenase in the presence and absence of indomethacin. This was done indirectly by determining the contractile response to arachidonic acid, the PG precursor (Figure 41). It has previously been well established that arachidonic acid elicits contraction from a resting gut through its conversion to PGE_1 and PGE_2.

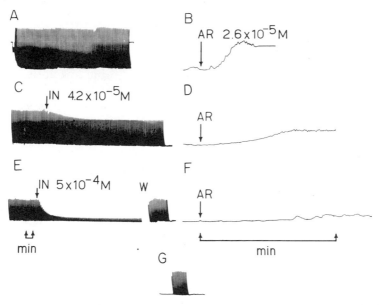

Figure 41. Effect of indomethacin (IN) on the response of the ileum to electrical stimulation compared with its effect on the response to arachidonic acid (AR). A and B. Control responses to electrical stimulation and arachidonic acid respectively. C. The effect of indomethacin (4.2 × 10^{-5} M) on the response to stimulation. D. The effect of indomethacin on the response to arachidonic acid. E. The effect of 5 × 10^{-4} M indomethacin on the response to stimulation and the reversibility by washing. F. The persistent effect of indomethacin after washout on the response to arachidonic acid. G. The response to stimulation following failure to respond to arachidonic acid. All drugs were added as in Figure 40. Final concentration is as indicated. In the figures showing responses to electrical stimulation, the chart speed was 5 mm/min; in those showing the responses to arachidonic acid, the chart speed was increased to 50 mm/min. [Gintzler and Musacchio]

Although indomethacin (4.2 × 10^{-5} M) has only a modest inhibitory effect on the response to electrical stimulation, it has a very substantial inhibitory effect on the contractile response to arachidonic acid (Figure 41C and D). Although the almost total inhibition of response to electrical stimulation caused by a higher concentration of indomethacin can be completely reversed by washing (Figure 41E), the inhibition of the response to arachidonic acid remains complete, indicating a permanent or semipermanent inhibition of PG synthesis (Figure 41F). Thus, even when the synthesis of PG is blocked, as demonstrated by the failure to respond to arachidonic acid, the gut can still respond to electrical stimulation (Figure 41G). This clearly indicates that the inhibitory effect of indomethacin on electrically induced contraction is independent of the inhibition of PG synthesis. It would thus appear that the mechanism by which PGE_2 interacts with morphine and norepinephrine is of a nonspecific nature and gives no insight into the possible neurochemistry of analgesia. In keeping with these findings, Simon reported that PGE_1 and PGE_2 do not show binding in the opiate receptor assay (Simon et al., 1973).

Musacchio discussed the interaction between serotonin and morphine in the guinea pig ileum (Gintzler and Musacchio, 1974). Because 5-HT is an endogenous neuronal constituent of the ileum, it is tempting to speculate that some interaction with the 5-HT system may play an essential role in the response of the ileum to morphine.

Serotonin increases the sensitivity of the ileum to morphine. If the preparation is initially treated with 3×10^{-7} M 5-HT and then allowed to recover from the inhibitory effects of this manipulation, the inhibition produced by 2×10^{-8} M morphine is increased from 45% to 100% (Gintzler and Musacchio, 1974). Following a number of washes, the response to morphine returns to control levels. Pretreatment with 5-HT also potentiates the inhibitory effects of nalorphine and methadone. This interaction between 5-HT and morphine is specific, because the inhibitory response to norepinephrine is unaffected by 5-HT, and norepinephrine itself has no effect on the inhibitory response to morphine. This is a particularly significant point, since norepinephrine, like morphine, is a potent inhibitor of both the spontaneous and electrically evoked release of acetylcholine in the guinea pig ileum. Thus, powerful inhibition of the gut of itself does not potentiate the inhibitory effects of morphine. Inhibiting the remaining response to electrical stimulation after the addition of 5-HT cannot be the basis for the potentiation. The implication of this interaction between the 5-HT system and opiates in terms of the ultimate mechanism of opiate action is not clear.

Since potentiation (synergism) between two compounds is an indication of the existence of a sequential effect in linear model enzyme systems (Black, 1963), the potentiation between 5-HT and morphine suggests that there might be a common biochemical pathway that mediates the effects of these drugs. The possibility that morphine may act in the gut and in the CNS by increasing the availability of 5-HT, and, in so doing, potentiate its inhibitory effects appeared unlikely, because on a number of occasions the ileum was insensitive to the inhibitory effects of 5-HT but still showed its usual sensitivity to the inhibitory effects of morphine. If morphine were acting simply by making more 5-HT available, the response to morphine should also be attenuated. Secondly, the ileum can be made refractory to the inhibitory effects of 5-HT by successively adding the drug while still in the presence of the previous addition. However, when the gut is made refractory to 5-HT, it still shows an augmented response to morphine. If morphine acts by releasing 5-HT or by blocking its reuptake, one would expect that when the gut no longer responds to the inhibitory effects of 5-HT, there would be no response to morphine.

Changes in Sensitivity to Neurotransmitters in the Opiate-Tolerant Myenteric Plexus: A. Goldstein

Goldstein reported the results of the investigations in his laboratory on the response of the isolated guinea pig ileum to 5-HT and morphine during morphine tolerance (Schulz and Goldstein, 1973). After guinea pigs are made tolerant and dependent by subcutaneous implantation of morphine pellets, the electrically stimulated muscle strips from these tolerant, dependent guinea pigs are also tolerant to the inhibitory action of morphine and show less sensitivity to the inhibitory actions of epinephrine, isoproterenol, and dopamine (Goldstein and Schulz, 1973). Their sensitivity to the spasmogenic action of acetylcholine was unchanged. In contrast, there is a large increase in sensitivity to 5-HT associated with morphine tolerance; strips from morphine-tolerant animals are about 10 times more sensitive to 5-HT. This degree of supersensitivity is very nearly the same as the degree of tolerance to morphine. Furthermore, after pellet removal, sensitivity to morphine and epinephrine increases at the same rate as the sensitivity to 5-HT decreases (Figure 42). Naloxone added to the bath before 5-HT challenge fails to affect control or tolerant strips. Exogenous 5-HT, like electrical stimulation, contracts the longitudinal muscle, which is blocked by atropine, suggesting that for both 5-HT and electrical stimulation, contraction is mediated by the release of acetylcholine.

Goldstein suggested that 5-HT is an excitatory transmitter in the myenteric plexus that elicits cholinergic stimulation of the muscle. This view is supported by Gershon's demonstration of terminals containing 5-HT in the plexus (Robinson and Gershon, 1971; Ross and Gershon, 1972). The serotonin-induced contraction of the longitudinal muscle is antagonized by morphine and norepinephrine, suggesting that the opiates, serotonin, and catecholamines influence the longitudinal

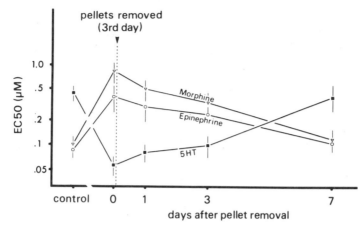

Figure 42. Changes in sensitivity of the myenteric plexus to neurotransmitters in the development of tolerance. Myenteric plexus/longitudinal muscle preparations from guinea pigs were tested in tissue bath at various times after removal of morphine pellets from the animals. Complete dose-response curves were established for inhibitory effects of morphine and epinephrine, and for excitatory effect of 5-HT. EC_{50} values are plotted, i.e., concentrations required for 50% inhibition of electrically induced twitch, or 50% of maximal stimulation of unstimulated preparation. [Schulz et al., 1974]

muscle through a common neural pathway. The acute effect of morphine could be to inhibit transmission at the excitatory synapse between the 5-HT terminals and the cholinergic neuron and thus decrease the output of acetylcholine and the twitch tension of the muscle. Goldstein hypothesized that an adrenergic neuron modulates transmission in an inhibitory manner at a synapse in the excitatory pathway, perhaps at the same serotonergic synapse through which morphine manifests its action. The finding that exogenous catechol-amines decrease the output of acetylcholine in this preparation strongly suggests a catecholamine action on some neural element of the plexus rather than a direct inhibitory action on the smooth muscle itself. This is consistent with histologic studies showing most adrenergic terminals ending very near ganglion cells in the plexus rather than penetrating into the smooth muscle layer (Jacobowitz, 1965; Costa and Furness, 1973). It is unclear whether morphine blocks postsynaptic 5-HT receptors or blocks transmission at the serotonergic synapse by mimicking the effects of catecholamines or by causing the release of catecholamines.

Goldstein reviewed the work of Gyang and Kosterlitz (1966), which showed that α- and β-adrenergic blockers do not interfere with the morphine effect in this preparation, indicating that morphine does not act by releasing norepinephrine or by combining with norepinephrine receptors. However, the possibility that morphine releases dopamine has not been ruled out.

Goldstein proposed that tolerance to morphine involves an increase in the number or in the intrinsic sensitivity of 5-HT receptors. Thus the normal function of the excitatory pathway would be restored in spite of the presence of morphine, and a greater concentration of morphine or catecholamines would be required for inhibition. Sensitization of the synapse would accomplish this regardless of whether morphine acted directly upon the 5-HT receptors or indirectly through the release of an inhibitory transmitter. Whether supersensitivity to 5-HT is due to increase in the number of 5-HT receptors or alteration of their properties is unknown.

In an attempt to localize the opiate receptor in different classes of neurons in the guinea pig ileum, Musacchio has treated guinea pigs with intravenous 6-hydroxydopamine, a drug that selectively lesions norepinephrine and dopamine neurons. The 6-hydroxydopamine treatment reduces tyrosine hydroxylase activity in the intestine by 90% (a measure of the destruction of catecholamine terminals) but fails to alter opiate receptor binding. Musacchio has also examined the guinea pig kidney, which possesses high levels of opiate receptor. Again, 6-hydroxydopamine injection, although reducing catecholamine terminals by approximately 90%, has no effect on opiate receptor binding.*

In the mouse vas deferens, morphine acts by decreasing the release of norepinephrine. If morphine acts directly on the postganglionic sympathetic nerve, 6-hydroxydopamine should abolish opiate receptor binding. Such experiments are currently being performed. Hughes felt that the opiate receptor in the mouse vas deferens is indeed localized in the nerve terminals of the sympathetic nerves and would be destroyed by 6-hydroxydopamine.

Musacchio also reported that adenosine triphosphate (ATP) potentiates the effects of morphine in the guinea pig ileum. The inhibition of contraction produced by ATP itself was not naloxone sensitive. Musacchio wondered whether morphine might act by release of ATP. However, direct measurement showed no efflux of ATP after morphine treatment.

As a logical extension of work characterizing the action of narcotics in the longitudinal muscle/myenteric plexus preparation, Dingledine, Goldstein, and Kendig (1974) have attempted to investigate

*J.M. Musacchio and G.L. Craviso, unpublished observations.

the neuronal basis for narcotic action on the myenteric plexus. Morphine inhibits the spontaneous electrical activity of many of the neurons studied, while serotonin elevates the firing rate of these cells. In most cases, units that did not respond to serotonin were not inhibited by morphine or levorphanol.

Morphine also prevents the increase in firing rate caused by serotonin. These effects of morphine were stereospecific and blocked by naloxone and are therefore considered to be specific opiate effects. Since morphine specifically affects the firing rate of neurons in the plexus, it is very unlikely that it acts directly on the terminals of the cholinergic motor neuron to depress acetylcholine release.

Interaction of Opiates and Neurotransmitters: E.L. Way

Way discussed the role of norepinephrine, dopamine, serotonin, and acetylcholine in morphine tolerance and dependence (Way, 1973). Catecholamines and acetylcholine do not seem to be involved in the development of tolerance. Evidence ruling out the catecholamines was obtained by injecting 6-hydroxydopamine intraventricularly to lesion selectively central catecholamine neurons. This 6-hydroxydopamine treatment reduced the analgesic effects of morphine. However, the treatment did not prevent the development of tolerance (Friedler et al., 1972; Bhargava et al., 1973). Elevation of brain acetylcholine by cholinesterase inhibition or lowering brain acetylcholine by inhibiting synthesis also failed to affect tolerance and dependence development (Bhargava and Way, 1972; Bhargava et al., 1975). By contrast, partial destruction of serotonin neurons in the brain by intraventricular injection of dihydroxytryptamine elicited a decrease in the development of tolerance to morphine analgesia. Animals pretreated with dihydroxytryptamine also seemed to become less physically dependent because they required a higher dose of naloxone to precipitate withdrawal signs (Figure 43) (Ho et al., 1973c).

A similar result was obtained by inhibiting 5-HT synthesis with *p*-chlorophenylalanine (PCPA). PCPA treatment reduced the development of tolerance to and dependence on morphine. After concurrent administration of PCPA with morphine, given repeatedly, the amount of naloxone needed to precipitate withdrawal jumping was roughly three times greater in the PCPA-treated than in the control group. Thus the sensitivity to naloxone, normally observed in addicted mice, was decreased after PCPA treatment (Shen et al., 1970; Ho et al., 1972b).

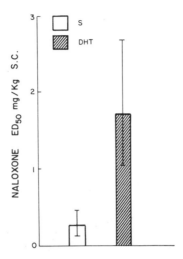

Figure 43. 5,6-Dihydroxytryptamine (DHT) inhibiton of physical dependence development on morphine. Decreased dependence is evidenced by the higher dose of naloxone (ED_{50}) required to precipitate withdrawal jumping in mice rendered dependent by morphine pellet implantation. The control mice (S) received isotonic saline in place of DHT. [Ho et al., 1973c]

In accordance with the conclusions of this study are experiments in which an increase in serotonin levels effected by the injection of its precursors, tryptophan or 5-hydroxytryptophan (5-HTP), in mice and rats accelerated the development of tolerance. The accelerating effect of tryptophan but not 5-HTP on tolerance development was prevented by PCPA (Figure 44). In addition to accelerating the rate of developing morphine tolerance, tryptophan enhanced the development of physical dependence in mice and rats during morphine pellet implantation. Animals treated with tryptophan became markedly more sensitive to naloxone after morphine pellet implantation (Ho et al., 1972d).

Way also reported that a single intravenous injection of cyclic AMP (10 mg/kg) accelerated the development of morphine tolerance and physical dependence (Ho et al., 1973a,b). This dose caused no mortality or overt toxic signs and had a surprisingly long duration of action. The analgesic action of morphine was also antagonized by this dose of cyclic AMP for at least 24 hours, but this appeared to be a separate or less specific action. The accelerating effect of cyclic AMP on the development of morphine tolerance and physical dependence was blocked by cycloheximide injected daily during the period of morphine pellet implantation (Figure 45). Though as yet he is unable to explain these results, Way notes with interest that cyclic AMP stimulates 5-HT

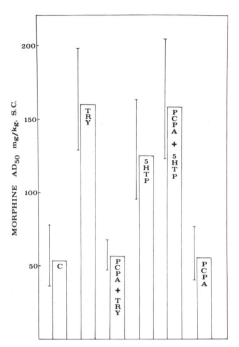

Figure 44. Tryptophan (TRY) and 5-hydroxytryptophan (5-HTP) enhancement of morphine tolerance development and effect of *p*-chlorophenylalanine (PCPA) on the response. Increased tolerance is evidenced by an elevation in the dose of morphine (AD_{50}) required to produce analgesia. All groups were rendered tolerant by morphine pellet implantation; the control group (C) received vehicle instead of test solution. [Ho et al., 1975]

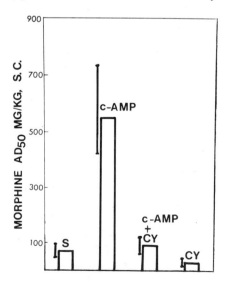

Figure 45. Cyclic 3′,5′-adenosine monophosphate (c-AMP) enhancement of morphine tolerance development and blockade of the response by cycloheximide (CY). Increased tolerance is evidenced by an elevation in the dose of morphine (AD_{50}) required to produce analgesia. Mice were rendered tolerant by morphine pellet implantation; the control group (S) received saline instead of the test solution. [Ho et al., 1973b]

turnover in the brain (Tagliamonte et al., 1971). Since tryptophan, like cyclic AMP, antagonizes morphine's antinociceptive action and accelerates the development of tolerance and physical dependence, a link may exist between the two substances.

In assessing the many diverse morphine abstinence signs, Way presented evidence suggesting that the stereotyped jumping behavior precipitated by naloxone in morphine-dependent mice and rats may depend on brain dopamine. During naloxone-precipitated withdrawal jumping, there was no change in the concentration of serotonin or norepinephrine in the brain. However there was a rapid elevation of dopamine levels of about 25% between 5 and 20 min after the injection of naloxone when jumping was maximal (Figure 46). The increase in dopamine occurred principally in the striatum and was not caused by jumping itself, because the increase was still present when jumping was prevented by curare. At a dose of naloxone that precipitated

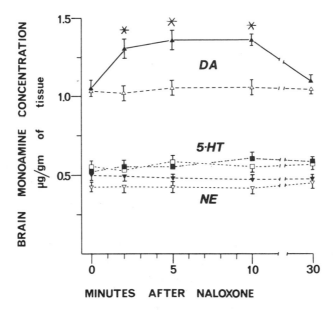

Figure 46. Brain monoamine levels in morphine-dependent mice during withdrawal jumping precipitated by naloxone. Naloxone (5 mg/kg injected subcutaneously) was given 6 h after removal of a morphine or placebo pellet implanted for 72 h. Black symbols denote morphine-implanted mice; white symbols, placebo-implanted mice. Each point represents the mean of three experiments using four mice each, except at 30 min, which represents the mean of a single experiment using eight mice. The vertical lines represent ± SEM. *, significantly different from placebo-implanted control, $p < .01$. DA = dopamine; 5-HT = serotonin; NE = norepinephrine. [Iwamoto et al., 1973]

withdrawal jumping in 50% of the mice, only those mice who jumped showed an increase in striatal dopamine levels. Pretreatment with the acetylcholinesterase inhibitor, physostigmine, which increases brain levels of acetylcholine, inhibited both the naloxone-precipitated withdrawal and the increase in striatal dopamine levels (Iwamoto et al., 1973). The administration of hemicholinium-3, which decreases acetylcholine synthesis, had the opposite effect and sensitized the morphine-dependent mice to naloxone (Bhargava et al., 1975). This suggests an interaction between cholinergic and dopaminergic mechanisms in the production of withdrawal jumping.

In attempting to determine the exact mechanism of the naloxone-induced increase in striatal dopamine levels, unilateral electrolytic nigrostriatal lesions were made in the rat, and the response of these animals to apomorphine, L-dopa, and amphetamine was studied according to the method of Andén and his co-workers (1966) (Figure 47). All three dopamine agonists cause rotation towards the lesioned side. In contrast, haloperidol or pimozide, dopamine receptor blocking agents, both caused rotation away from the lesioned side. In

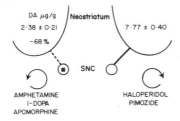

Figure 47. Turning response to dopamine agonists (*left*) and antagonists (*right*) in the rat after electrolytic coagulation of the left substantia nigra (SNC). Dopamine (DA) levels in the neostriatum of the lesioned and the intact side are also given. [After Andén et al., 1966]

morphine-dependent animals, naloxone also caused rotation away from the lesioned side, which can be reversed by apomorphine but not by haloperidol. Apomorphine also suppressed other precipitated withdrawal signs, whereas haloperidol did not. Way concluded that the release of dopamine was suddenly decreased in precipitated withdrawal, possibly as a consequence of decreased neuronal activity. This would explain the rapid increase in striatal dopamine levels after naloxone administration. The increase in striatal dopamine levels was accompanied by an increase in the acid metabolites of dopamine, homovanillic acid and dihydroxyphenylacetic acid (Tseng et al., 1974). Perhaps acute administration of morphine enhances dopamine utilization, and dopamine turnover increases as a compensatory response. Tolerance develops to these effects, and the availability of dopamine becomes dependent on the presence of morphine. In the dependent state, precipitation of withdrawal with naloxone may decrease dopamine neuronal firing and produce an opposite effect.

Creese emphasized the problem of determining whether modifications of behavioral responses elicited in precipitated withdrawal are primary to the morphine abstinence syndrome or if manipulations of certain neurotransmitter systems serve only to disrupt an efferent motor component of the response, which is determined on a different level. For example, because the nigrostriatal dopamine pathway is part of the extrapyramidal motor system, it might be expected that any manipulation of dopamine would affect the expression of overt motor behavior without necessarily implying that the dopamine system was the primary site of opiate action. Creese also commented on the fact that the unilateral nigrostriatal lesions made by Way were incomplete. Ungerstedt (1971a,b) has shown that with a complete unilateral nigrostriatal lesion, amphetamine and apomorphine are distinguished from each other by causing rotation in opposite directions, reflecting a different mechanism of action within the dopamine system. Amphetamine causes a release of endogenous dopamine on the intact side, and apomorphine stimulates to a greater extent the denervated receptors on the lesioned side. Because apomorphine and amphetamine caused rotation in the same direction in Way's preparation, complex interactions between supersensitive receptors and the remaining intact dopamine neurons on the lesioned side were prominent. In fact, in the apomorphine-treated rat, it appeared that apomorphine had more effect on the intact striatum. Way replied that Ungerstedt used 6-hydroxydopamine instead of electrolytic coagulation to make a lesion, and the response to apomorphine is different in the two preparations. However, contralateral turning was obtained in dependent animals with both methods when naloxone was injected.

Herz also pointed out that, according to Way's results, haloperidol, which blocks dopamine receptors, should precipitate jumping if Way's conclusion suggesting that naloxone inhibits dopamine release is correct. In fact, haloperidol inhibits the expression of withdrawal symptoms. Way answered that morphine and haloperidol both produce catalepsy in naive animals by reducing dopamine activity, but that their sites of action appear to differ and that in his laboratory haloperidol did not affect precipitated withdrawal. Herz found that apomorphine enhanced jumping during precipitated withdrawal, whereas apomorphine inhibited jumping in Way's preparation.

Snyder suggested that this discrepancy may be more apparent than real. Ungerstedt* has found that in naive animals low doses of apomorphine inhibit motor activity, whereas higher doses stimulate it. This is explained elegantly by the hypothesis of Bunney and Aghajanian (1975) that presynaptic dopamine receptors on the surface of dopamine neurons are more sensitive to dopamine and apomorphine than the postsynaptic receptors. These presynaptic receptors respond to dopamine and apomorphine by an inhibition of dopamine release and hence a decrease in dopaminergic activity. By contrast, at the postsynaptic receptor, apomorphine stimulates dopamine receptors, enhancing the dopamine-like behavior. If the presynaptic receptor is more sensitive to dopamine and apomorphine than the postsynaptic receptor, it is perfectly reasonable for low doses of apomorphine to inhibit motor activity and high doses to stimulate stereotyped motor behavior. However, Creese pointed out that the discrepancy appeared not at high doses of apomorphine, for which Way and Herz both reported a decrease in withdrawal signs, but at somewhat lower doses. Way observed a decrease in abstinence signs at 3 mg/kg apomorphine, and Herz found an increase in precipitated withdrawal jumping at 2.5 mg/kg apomorphine. Such results emphasize the problem of interpreting drug interaction studies in which differences in the degree of dependence or in the time interval between drug administration and naloxone-precipitated withdrawal and the nonspecificity of a drug's action can all influence the emergent behaviors.

Significance of Catecholamines in Opiate Dependence and Withdrawal: A. Herz

Herz presented data on the role of catecholaminergic mechanisms in the expression of the morphine abstinence syndrome and in the development of morphine dependence in rats. The effect of drugs affecting catecholaminergic mechanisms on various signs of precipitated morphine withdrawal was studied in rats that had developed a medium degree of dependence by pellet implantation (6 pellets within 10 days). Low doses of d-amphetamine, cocaine, and L-dopa given shortly before precipitating withdrawal induced a dose-dependent increase of "dominant" withdrawal signs such as jumping, and a decrease of "recessive" signs such as wet dog shaking (Table 13); signs such as diarrhea and

*U. Ungerstedt, personal communication.

TABLE 13

Modification of Precipitated Withdrawal in the Rat by Pretreatment with Drugs,
Increased Dependence, or Increased Dosage of Antagonist [Herz]

	Jumping (flying)	Teeth chattering	Wet dog shaking	Writhing	Ptosis	Eye twitches	Rhinorrhea	Diarrhea
d-Amphetamine (0.5–2.0 mg/kg)	↑	↑	↓	±	↓	±	↑	↓
Cocaine (5.0–10.0 mg/kg)	↑	±	↓	±	↓	±	↑	(↓)
L-Dopa + Ro 4-4602 (100.0 mg/kg)	↑	±	↓	±	↓	↑	(↑)	↓
Apomorphine (1.0–2.5 mg/kg)	↑	(↑)	±	±	↓	(↑)	±	↓
Desipramine (2.5–20.0 mg/kg)	↑	(↑)	↓	±	↓	↑	±	↓
α-Methylparatyrosine (420 mg/kg)	↓	±	↓	↑	±	↓	±	±
FLA-63 (60 mg/kg)	↓	↓	↓	(↑)	±	±	±	↓
Increase in dependence (6/10 → 24/9 groups 1 mg/kg levallorphan)	↑	(↑)	↑	±	±	↑	↑	↓
Increase in antagonist (24/9 groups 1.0 → 10.0 mg/kg levallorphan)	↓	±	±	±	↓	(↑)	↑	↓

↑ increase; ↓ decrease; ± equivocal results. Arrows in parentheses indicate trends not statistically significant. The dose range considered of each drug is given in parentheses. Rhinorrhea also stands for lacrimation and salivation.

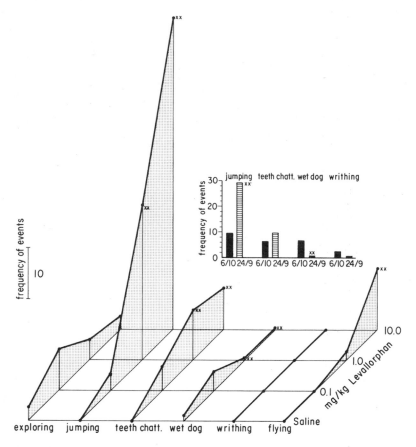

Figure 48. Effect of precipitating morphine withdrawal with increasing doses of levallorphan in highly dependent rats; 24 morphine pellets were implanted subcutaneously within 9 days. On the 9th day withdrawal was precipitated with increasing doses of levallorphan. *Insert:* Comparison of withdrawal syndrome in rats with a medium (6/10) and a high (24/9) degree of dependence. Withdrawal was precipitated by levallorphan 1 mg/kg intraperitoneally. [Herz]

ptosis decreased, whereas rhinorrhea, lacrimation, and salivation increased. Qualitatively, a very similar "shift" in signs occurred when withdrawal was precipitated by the same dose of antagonist (1 mg/kg levallorphan) in highly dependent rats and/or was precipitated by high doses of the antagonist (Figure 48). These drugs therefore seem to potentiate withdrawal in spite of the fact that some signs are reduced.

Selective activation of noradrenergic mechanisms by desipramine had a strong potentiating effect (Figure 49). In the case of stimulation of dopaminergic mechanisms by apomorphine, this potentiating effect was much weaker and restricted to a limited dose range (2

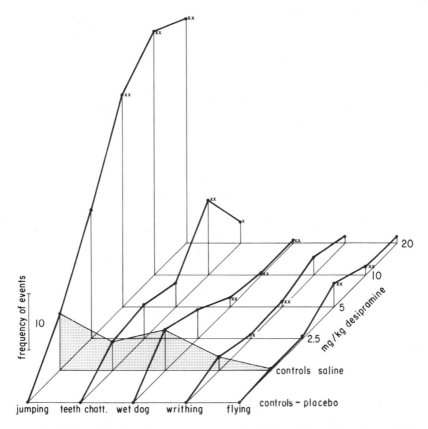

Figure 49. Effect of desipramine on some counted withdrawal signs of morphine withdrawal precipitated by levallorphan. Six morphine pellets were implanted within 10 days; on the 10th day desipramine was injected intraperitoneally at a dose ranging between 2.5 and 20 mg/kg, 30 min before levallorphan 1 mg/kg. x, p < 0.05; xx, p < 0.01 in respect to dependent controls. [Herz]

to 5 mg/kg). At higher doses jumping was decreased. It is supposed that the strong stereotyped behavior obvious at the higher doses of apomorphine, *d*-amphetamine, and cocaine suppresses other motor behaviors.

It appears that both brain dopamine and norepinephrine are involved in the manifestation of withdrawal, but norepinephrine is more important.

The significance of catecholamines for the development of morphine dependence was studied in experiments in which chronic depletion of the brain catecholamines was induced by means of α-methylparatyrosine (Figure 50).

122

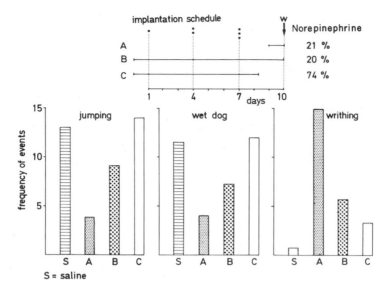

Figure 50. Changes in counted withdrawal signs after pretreatment with α-methylparatyrosine (AMPT) at 3 different administration schedules. Schedule A: 420 mg/kg (6 portions) during the last 24 h before withdrawal; schedule B: 300 mg/kg/day (6 portions) of AMPT starting 24 h before first implantation of pellets and discontinuing 4 h before withdrawal; schedule C: AMPT injections as under B, but discontinuing 40 h before withdrawal. The rats had received 6 morphine pellets (75 mg) within 10 days; withdrawal was precipitated by levallorphan 1 mg/kg intramuscularly. [Bläsig]

In schedule A, α-methylparatyrosine (AMPT) was given only during the last 2 days of the 10-day implantation period. The 80% decline in brain norepinephrine levels was accompanied by a strong reduction in withdrawal intensity (low jumping, high writhing; see also Table 13). This is consistent with the opposite effects obtained with catecholaminergic stimulants. In schedule B, AMPT was given during the whole implantation period, also producing an 80% depletion in norepinephrine. In this case, inhibition of withdrawal was significantly reduced in comparison to schedule A. In schedule C, AMPT treatment was given during the first 8 days of exposure to morphine and then was terminated, allowing catecholamine synthesis to be reinstated. By the time of levallorphan-precipitated withdrawal, norepinephrine was only 30% depleted. In this case a quite normal withdrawal pattern was observed. From this one might conclude that catecholamines are not essential for the development of morphine dependence. However, the fact that prolonged treatment with AMPT tended to produce a pattern more closely approximating that seen in normal withdrawal indicates

development of supersensitivity of catecholamine receptors that antagonize the influence of catecholamine depletion. Therefore, a definitive
answer to whether catecholamines are involved in the mechanisms
leading to physical dependence on morphine cannot be given, although
it is improbable that they are very important.

124

VI. ADDICTION

Background

Himmelsbach (1941) carefully examined the morphine abstinence syndrome in patients withdrawn from opiates at the Public
Health Service Hospital in Lexington, Kentucky. His is the most
complete systematic clinical description of opiate withdrawal. His
scoring system for the signs of opiate withdrawal excludes drug-craving
or drug-seeking behavior and concentrates on the physiological signs of
withdrawal. Himmelsbach later related this scoring system to the degree
of opiate dependence as measured by the total daily dose of morphine
(Andrews and Himmelsbach, 1944). The study was conducted with the
cooperation of opiate-dependent patients who were stabilized upon
admission to the hospital with doses of morphine sufficient to prevent
withdrawal (Table 14). At the termination of maintenance therapy, the

TABLE 14

Stabilization Dose Range for 127 Patients
[Modified from Andrews and Himmelsbach, 1944]

Group (number)	Dose range (mg morphine)	Average dose (mg morphine)
13	400 to 500	407
14	300 to 350	302
31	200 to 280	212
21	150 to 180	160
19	100 to 140	118
13	75 to 90	80
11	60	60
5	40	40

morphine was abruptly withdrawn and average abstinence syndrome
intensity (ASI) was determined for the first 7 days after withdrawal.
Average daily abstinence scores were then plotted against the stabilization dose, resulting in a hyperbolic curve (Figure 51).

If one plots these data using the logarithm of the dose, the
classic sigmoid-shaped curve of dose-response curves results. It has been
speculated that these curves indicate the saturation of opiate receptors
in man. Many studies have measured various subjective and physiolog-

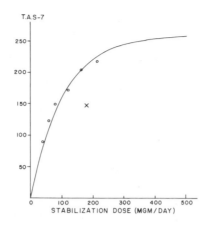

Figure 51. The T.A.S.-7 dose relationship. The average abstinence syndrome intensity (ASI) per day was determined for each group for the first 7 days of abstinence. The plotted points were connected by straight lines, and the area under each curve was measured with a planimeter. These areas were converted into point-days and then became measures of the total abstinence syndrome for 7 days (T.A.S.-7). ○ = experimental points; × = a group of 9 patients who received a rapid reduction treatment. [Andrews and Himmelsbach, 1944]

ical parameters after single-dose administration of opiates in nondependent subjects. These parameters often show a linear relationship to log dose. Higher doses that might show a decrease in slope are generally not administered because of the possibility of toxic opiate effects. The only data in man that appear to show saturation are Himmelsbach's plots of ASI against stabilization dose. Of interest in this speculation is the group of drugs termed "partial agonists" in Chapter III, "Agonist-Antagonist Interactions" (see also Jasinski et al., 1971). These opiate-like drugs exhibit pure opiate-like effects in single doses, and when administered chronically they produce physical dependence indistinguishable qualitatively from that of morphine. Partial agonists will support morphine dependence in subjects stabilized on 60 mg morphine/day but will precipitate abstinence in subjects dependent on 240 mg morphine/day. Jasinski and his colleagues (1971) have proposed that these opiate-like drugs have lower intrinsic activity than morphine. Thus they have been termed "partial agonists."

Partial agonists behave like antagonists in animal studies, precipitating withdrawal in dependent primates. Perhaps if the studies had been conducted on animals stabilized on different daily doses, results similar to those from human data would have been observed.

Clinical Phenomenology of Addiction:
W.R. Martin

Martin has studied opiate withdrawal in man employing a modified Himmelsbach scoring system (Table 15). He emphasized that the Himmelsbach scoring system lists the signs of withdrawal beginning with the early or minimal signs, such as yawning, lacrimation, rhinorrhea, and perspiration, and progressing to signs seen in more intense withdrawal or later in the time course of withdrawal, such as goose flesh, tremor, restlessness, and emesis.

TABLE 15

Source of Points for Abstinence Scores
[Martin, 1966; Jasinski et al., 1967]

Sign	Point value
Yawning	1
Lacrimation	1
Rhinorrhea	1
Perspiration	1
Goose flesh	3
Tremor	3
Restlessness	5
Emesis	5
Each 0.1 mm pupil dilation	1
Each increase in respiratory rate	1
Each 2 mm increase in systolic blood pressure	1
Each 0.1°C rise in body temperature	1

Each withdrawal sign has been given a point value; after the observation period, the points are added up to form the abstinence score.

Martin described the phenomenology of a cycle of morphine dependence as studied in opiate-experienced subjects (Martin and Jasinski, 1969). These subjects had used opiates for 14 to 20 years but had not been dependent for at least 5 months prior to the study. The study lasted 74 weeks, including a drug-free period or control period of 7 weeks, chronic administration of morphine for 31 weeks (stabilizing at 240 mg morphine/day by the 5th week), slow withdrawal of morphine over a 3-week period, and follow-up observations for 31 weeks.

After opiate administration, a slight increase in average systolic and diastolic blood pressure along with a less consistent increase in pulse rate was observed (Figure 52). Body temperature was increased

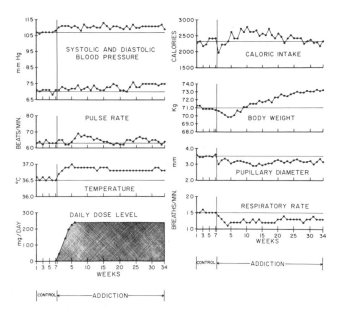

Figure 52. The effects of chronic administration of morphine on clinical variables. Each point represents the weekly mean A.M. observations for 7 subjects. The horizontal line represents the mean of control determinations for 7 subjects. [Martin and Jasinski, 1969]

by about 0.5°C. There was an initial decrease in caloric intake that returned to normal in a few weeks. Body weight fell by about 1 kg over 4 weeks but then returned to normal and increased thereafter.

The respiratory rate and pupillary diameter remained slightly depressed during a cycle of dependence. There was, however, a marked tolerance to the respiratory-depressing and pupillary-constricting effects of morphine; additional doses of morphine had little effect on these parameters. During the above study, Martin gave the subjects (who were receiving 60 mg of morphine 4 times/day) a single dose of 120 mg of morphine (twice the stabilizing dose). Employing measurements of respiratory center sensitivity to carbon dioxide by the rebreathing technique only, a minimal further decrease in sensitivity was observed (Martin et al., 1968), and there was very little change in pupil size.

These results were interpreted using the redundancy theory of tolerance and dependence. Martin (1970) has postulated that there may be two systems subserving respiratory drive. One is blocked completely by 240 mg of morphine/day. The other, which is largely insensitive to opiates, remains intact and is not depressed by morphine. Hypertrophy of this morphine-insensitive system may account for hypersensitivity of the carbon dioxide center to hypercapnic stimulation seen after

128

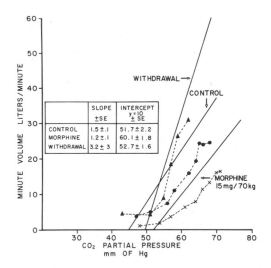

Figure 53. Mean calculated regression lines for $pACO_2$-VA (carbon dioxide partial pressure-alveolar ventilation) response curves obtained during the control period, after 15 mg/70 kg of morphine, and during early withdrawal in subjects dependent on 240 mg/day of morphine. The means for each parameter were determined from values obtained in 7 subjects. There was great variability in the first and last points of the response curves. The top of the regression lines represents the maximum VA obtained. A control (●), a 15 mg/70 kg dose of morphine (×), and a withdrawal (▲) $pACO_2$-VA response of one subject are presented to further illustrate these changes. [Martin et al., 1968]

withdrawal, when both this system and the formerly morphine-depressed system act together. Evidence for this is consistent with a change in the intercept and slope of the respiratory center response to hypercapnia in which the line was shifted to the left and its slope increased (Figure 53 and Table 16).

Further depression of respiratory center sensitivity to carbon dioxide in protracted abstinence may then be explained by a compensatory inactivation of the morphine-insensitive system during the first 7 weeks of (early) abstinence. Although this explanation fits the data described above, there is no critical experimental evidence to support it.

Martin presented a graph illustrating changes in physiological parameters during the early abstinence period followed by changes observed after the seventh to tenth week of withdrawal (Figure 54). These later changes, termed "protracted abstinence," consist of decreases in pulse rate, body temperature, appetite and body weight, pupillary size, sensitivity of the respiratory center to carbon dioxide, and a slight decrease in blood pressure. Physical dependence can be

TABLE 16

The Effect of Early (Primary) Abstinence Determined During
the Early Part of Stabilization (2 Months of Addiction) and
During the Period of Dose Reduction [Martin et al., 1968]

	Slope ± SE	Intercept (Y = 10 ± SE)
Control	1.5 ± 0.1	51.7 ± 2.2
Primary abstinence		
early withdrawal	3.2 ± 0.3*	52.7 ± 1.6
dose reduction	2.1 ± 0.3*	45.3 ± 1.4*

One patient using methadone was withdrawn and tested 2 days after his last dose of methadone. Withdrawal means and standard errors were calculated from data obtained 19 h after the last dose of morphine except for the dose reduction determination made in the patient withdrawn on methadone.
*Significantly different from control determination at the p < .05 level using a paired replicate analysis.

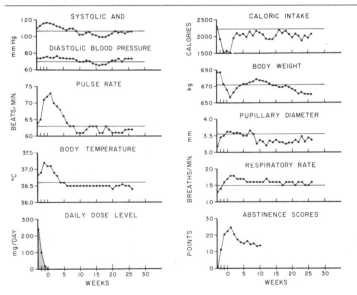

Figure 54. Changes seen during early and protracted abstinence. Each point represents the mean weekly A.M. values for 6 subjects. The first point of each curve represents the mean value for the last 7 weeks of addiction. The horizontal line represents the mean control value for the 6 subjects. One subject was withdrawn from the study near the end of the chronic intoxication phase because of episodes of acute cholecystitis. [Martin and Jasinski, 1969]

obtained with cyclazocine and nalorphine as well as with morphine. However, the abstinence syndrome seen with these drugs is different from morphine abstinence.

TABLE 17

The Relative Percentage and Rank of Various Sources of Himmelsbach Points
for Morphine, Cyclazocine, and Nalorphine Abstinence Syndromes
[Martin and Gorodetzky, 1965]

Source of Points	Morphine		Cyclazocine		Nalorphine	
	% of total points	Rank	% of total points	Rank	% of total points	Rank
+ Signs	4.4	6	12.8	4	11.0	3
++ Signs	9.3	5	16.7	2	3.8	7
Caloric intake	1.9	8	5.5	6	6.7	6
Restlessness	0.8	9	0	9	1.1	8
Emesis	2.8	7	0.7	8	0	9
Fever	12.3	3	33.9	1	35.8	1
Hyperpnea	31.1	1	11.1	5	10.8	4
Systolic blood pressure	25.5	2	3.1	7	9.9	5
Weight loss	11.5	4	15.8	3	20.9	2

The values for morphine and cyclazocine have been previously reported by Martin and his co-workers (1965). The values for nalorphine were calculated from data obtained from 7 experimental subjects. Spearman correlation coefficients (Snedecor, 1956) for the various conditions are: morphine X cyclazocine = .47 (<.05); morphine X nalorphine = .60 (<.05); cyclazocine X nalorphine = .72 (<.05). Values in parentheses indicate the level of significance for the correlations.

The nalorphine and cyclazocine abstinence syndromes included all the signs seen after morphine withdrawal and therefore grossly resembled morphine abstinence. However, as illustrated in Table 17, the rank order of signs was markedly changed. Moreover, withdrawal from cyclazocine and nalorphine was not accompanied by drug-craving or drug-seeking behavior (Martin and Gorodetzky, 1965; Martin et al., 1965). Although tolerance developed to the subjective and physiological effects of cyclazocine and nalorphine, tolerance did not develop to their ability to antagonize the effects of other opiates.

Does the rank order of signs seen after cyclazocine and nalorphine withdrawal relate to their lower morphine-like agonist activity? If so, should one see a similar symptom rank order with morphine dependence at low doses? To resolve these questions, Martin reviewed the unpublished work of E.G. Williams (Table 18). Williams gave morphine in different doses for various time durations. Martin reevaluated these data to determine whether the pattern of abstinence symptoms differs with the different treatment regimens. These treat-

TABLE 18

Spearman Rank Correlation Coefficients Between Sources of Himmelsbach
Abstinence Points for Various Morphine Addiction Cycles [Martin, 1966]

	10 mg qid 7 D	10 mg qid 10 D	10 mg qid 30 D	15 mg qid 10 D	15 mg qid 30 D	20 mg qid 30 D
10 mg qid 7 D						
10 mg qid 10 D	0.98					
10 mg qid 30 D	0.93	0.91				
15 mg qid 10 D	0.93	0.94	0.88			
15 mg qid 30 D	0.95	0.94	0.98	0.94		
20 mg qid 30 D	0.84	0.88	0.92	0.92	0.92	
60 mg qid 20 D	0.95	0.96	0.85	0.97	0.91	0.85

The dose levels indicated in the first 6 studies were held constant throughout the time period
indicated. Data used in the calculations are from unpublished studies of E.G. Williams. A
rapidly accelerating dose schedule was employed in the 7th study, and the dose level indicated
is the stabilization dose. The studies from which these data were obtained have been previously
reported (Fraser et al., 1961).

ments ranged from 10 mg 4 times/day for 7 days to 60 mg 4 times/day
for 20 days. He showed that the pattern of withdrawal is the same for
all of these treatment regimens, although the intensity varies.

Martin described a study in which subjects were given methadone chronically; a stabilization dose of 100 mg/day was achieved over
a 6-week period, maintained for 14 weeks, and the drug was then
withdrawn. While on methadone, systolic and diastolic blood pressure
were decreased as was pulse rate, while body temperature increased,
pupillary diameter and respiratory rate decreased, and the subjects
initially felt euphoric. Upon withdrawal, blood pressure, pulse rate, and
body temperature rose, pupil size and respiratory rate increased, and
Himmelsbach scores indicated pronounced withdrawal with a longer
duration than occurs with morphine. A protracted abstinence syndrome
was also observed after methadone withdrawal (Figure 55) (Martin
et al., 1973b). Statistical analysis of the rank order of the abstinence
syndrome with methadone and morphine showed marked similarities
(Table 19).

Changes in feeling state were prominent effects of chronic
opiate administration. Using the Minnesota Multiphasic Personality
Inventory (MMPI) during the tenth week of addiction to methadone,
there was an increase of the schizophrenia (Sc) and hypochondriasis
(Hy) scores that continued during the abstinence period (Table 20).
This does not mean that the individuals were schizophrenic; rather it
signifies social withdrawal and excessive concern with body function.

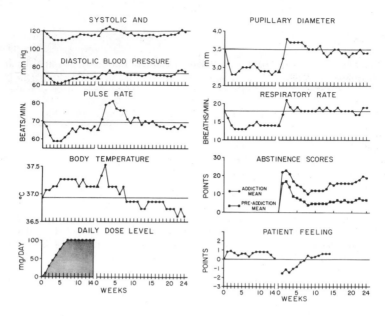

Figure 55. Changes in physiological indices and intensity of abstinence and feeling state during cycle of methadone dependence. Horizontal line in each graph represents mean of control observations made 3 times daily (6 A.M., 12 noon, and 6 P.M.) for 42 days in 5 patients. Each point represents mean weekly value. ▲ = mean of observations obtained during last 3 weeks of addiction cycle. [Martin et al., 1973b]

TABLE 19

The Relative Percentage and Rank of Sources of Himmelsbach Points for the Morphine and Methadone Abstinence Syndromes [Martin]

Source of Points	Morphine		Methadone	
	% of total points	Rank	% of total points	Rank
+ Signs	4.4	6	14.7	4
++ Signs	9.3	5	20.6	1
Caloric intake	1.9	8	3.4	7
Restlessness	0.8	9	2.2	9
Emesis	2.8	7	3.0	8
Fever	12.3	3	11.9	5
Hyperpnea	31.1	1	18.2	2
Systolic blood pressure	25.5	2	17.6	3
Weight loss	11.5	4	8.4	6

Spearman rank order correlation coefficient = .733 (p < .05). The data on morphine are a composite of studies done by E.G. Williams and H.F. Fraser at the Addiction Research Center.

TABLE 20

MMPI Scale Scores Through a Cycle of Methadone Dependence
[Martin et al, 1973b]

Scale	Control	Addiction (week)			Withdrawal (week)				
		1	4	10	4	8	12	16	20
N	5	5	5	5	4	5	5	4	4
L	50	51	51	50	47	53	49	54	51
F	63	65	61	67	68	62	65	75	70
K	55	56	56	53	52	56	56	60	57
Hs	54	56	60	71*	75*	58	53	61	53
D	65	60	65	74	86	70	69	70	64
Hy	53	56	59*	66*	71*	62†	57	66	58
Pd	78	78	80	76	86	81	83	88	80
Mf	65	62	62	65	70	66	64	66	68
Pa	60	66	63	60	67	61	63	64	58
Pt	59	60	60	63	70	66	68	68	64
Sc	62	67	64	70†	74*	68	70	77*	74*
Ma	68	67	68	65	70	69	66	68	72
Si	51	50	51	54	56	51	55	52	49

N = number of subjects. One patient participating in this study was semiliterate and could not independently complete the questionnaire; one patient refused to complete the test 4 weeks following withdrawal; another patient was transferred and did not complete the MMPI at the 16th and 20th weeks of withdrawal.
*$p < 0.1$ using a paired "T" test.
†$p < 0.05$ using a paired "T" test.

Measured by the ARCI (Haertzen, 1966), chronic administration of methadone leads to elevation of the pentobarbital-chlorpromazine-alcohol group scale and other scales that indicate lethargy, sedation, weakness, and decreased motivation (Table 21), in contrast to the euphorogenic effects seen with single doses of methadone (as indicated by elevation of the morphine-benzedrine group scale).

Martin feels that these findings, along with the changes on the MMPI and other personality variables, indicate a state of slight hypophoria as the length of opiate-dependence increases. This hypophoria involves an increase in the prevalence of negative feeling states and a decrease in positive feelings. This state of hypophoria increases markedly upon methadone withdrawal and is prominent for at least 20 weeks after withdrawal.

Hypophoria, the term preferred by Martin, is distinguished from depression in that hypophoria is characterized primarily by feelings of

134

TABLE 21

Addiction Research Center Inventory Scale Scores Through
a Cycle of Methadone Dependence [Martin et al., 1973b]

Scale	Control	Addiction (week)		Withdrawal (week)	
		1	4 and 10 (mean)	4	8, 12, 16, and 20 (mean)
General drug effect	48	62	61	80†	53
Negative feeling scales					
Pentobarbital-chlorpromazine-alcohol group	43	49	55*	73†	47
Weak	42	43	51	72†	47
Tired	44	53	61†	73†	47 (20)
Chlorpromazine specific	40	45	58†	76†	49
Narcotic antagonist	43	50	52	76	50†
Social withdrawal	56	57	56	58†	61
Critical	54	51	48†	42†	48 (20)
Chronic opiate	52	60	69†	68	53
Positive feeling scales					
Morphine-benzedrine group	55	55	53	38*	48 (20)
Popularity	47	37†	36†	21	36 (12,16,20)
Efficiency	58	54	48†	24†	51 (12,20)
Competitive	45	42	40	23†	36
Self-control	43	40	41	32	41 (16)
Benzedrine group	61	57	52†	29†	55 (20)
Withdrawal scales					
Alcohol withdrawal specific	45	46	50	68†	47
Drunk	44	52	52	68†	44
Weak opiate withdrawal	44	46	58†	73†	47
Severe opiate withdrawal	46	50	55	80†	50

Number of subjects is the same as in Table 20. Figures in parentheses indicate weeks mean score
significantly different from control.
*p < 0.1.
†p < 0.05.

being unpopular and by a poor self-image. The subjects have a poor
self-image, not because they think they are unworthy, but because they
feel other people do not like them. Snyder suggested that they may be
a little paranoid. Martin indicated that this feeling state lacks the weight
loss and sleep disturbance seen in endogenous depression. It should be
noted that these observations were made on subjects during a cycle of
opiate dependence in an experimental setting; all subjects were federal
prisoners confined to the housing and grounds of the Addiction
Research Center.

VII. FUTURE RESEARCH: DISCUSSION REVIEW

L.L. Iversen

Iversen summarized the proceedings of the Work Session, organizing them into several major categories. First in importance in terms of recent progress is our improved understanding of the interaction of the opiate drugs with their recognition or receptor sites. The demonstration that an endogenous ligand for the opiate receptor may exist in brain is also a discovery of crucial importance. The many events intervening in the "black box" between the CNS receptor sites and pharmacological effects are far more elusive. Equally perplexing are the mechanisms underlying tolerance and physical dependence.

In studies of the molecular pharmacology of opiate receptors, an important question for future research concerns the relationship of the cerebroside sulfate binding of opiates described by Loh to the opiate receptor in intact tissue. Since cerebroside sulfate preparations do bind opiates with high affinity, and this in turn shows some correlation with pharmacological potency, cerebrosides may be related in some way to the opiate receptors. One possibility, Iversen suggested, is that a cerebroside may be the "prosthetic group" of the opiate receptor, as heme is related to globin in hemoglobin function.

The distribution of the receptors in the brain is clearly important in understanding the pharmacological actions of opiates. There seems to be an excellent correlation of the distribution of biochemically assayed receptor sites with areas known to be significant for the perception of pain. The actions of sodium on opiate binding described by Snyder's group suggest that these receptors may be located on the external surfaces of cells where they would normally be exposed to relatively high sodium-ion concentrations. Snyder and his collaborators have shown synaptic membrane fractions to be the most enriched in receptor binding sites. The receptor could be located on the membranes of neuron cell bodies as well as on nerve terminals, because both would be included in synaptic membrane fractions.

Iversen speculated about the significance of the endogenous morphine-like substance discovered by Hughes and by Terenius and recently examined by Pasternak and Snyder. One might assume that this substance behaves like a neurotransmitter, and that opiates interact with the receptor sites for this hypothetical transmitter substance.

The focus of opiate research on such a postsynaptic receptor contrasts sharply with research on catecholamines and other CNS transmitters, where much effort has been expended on the study of presynaptic mechanisms. Certain drugs, such as 8-oxocyclazocines and N-methylfurylnorcyclazocines described by Kosterlitz, may well act by affecting the presynaptic disposition of the endogenous ligand. Once the endogenous compound is identified, there are a multitude of pharmacological approaches possible for manipulating its synaptic functions. One might develop inhibitors of synthesis, compounds that could act as false transmitters for the substance, and drugs that might enhance its release or reuptake (should it be inactivated at synapses by reuptake).

Of all the aspects of opiate pharmacology, the one that remains most enigmatic is the basis of tolerance and dependence. So far, no definitive information relating changes in opiate receptor biochemistry to addiction has been obtained. Perhaps the development of an irreversible label for the receptor would shed light on this problem. One would then be able to measure the rate of turnover of the opiate receptor molecule itself. Perhaps alterations in the rate of receptor turnover underlie the process of addiction, although it is quite conceivable that long-term changes of some other, as yet obscure nature are involved.

VIII. A MODEL OF OPIATE RECEPTOR FUNCTION WITH IMPLICATIONS FOR A THEORY OF ADDICTION

An Essay by S.H. Snyder

One of the aims of the Work Session was to integrate what is known of opiate pharmacology with new information about the opiate receptor. During the meeting, data were presented consistent with an allosteric model of opiate receptor function that would explain the differential influences of sodium on receptor binding of agonists and antagonists and might explain their pharmacological effects. This essay summarizes key features of this model (Pert and Snyder, 1974), offers new experimental evidence in its support, and applies the model toward a novel theory of the addictive process.

The influence of sodium upon opiate receptor binding is so specific and well correlated with the pharmacology of these drugs that it appears to represent an integral feature of opiate receptor function. Sodium produces proportionate increases and decreases respectively in the amount of antagonist and agonist binding. It is as if sodium increases the number of antagonist receptors and decreases the number of agonist receptors. However, because opiate agonists and antagonists are so similar chemically, it seems more reasonable to postulate that both drugs bind to the same receptor but that the opiate binding site can vary as the receptor is transformed back and forth between two different conformations (Figure 56). Sodium, which is responsible for the transition between the "sodium" or "antagonist" state of the receptor and the "no-sodium" or "agonist" state, differs in structure from the opiates and so, presumably, acts at an allosteric site. In our model, the binding of sodium by the receptor fixes the receptor in the antagonist conformation for which antagonists have a high and agonists

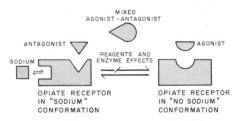

Figure 56. A model of opiate receptor function. [Pert and Snyder, 1974; Pasternak et al., 1975]

a very low affinity. Agonists would have substantial affinity for the agonist or no-sodium form of the receptor, whereas antagonists would have a reduced affinity for the no-sodium state. Mixed agonist-antagonists would have intermediate affinities for the two forms.

Typical morphine effects such as analgesia and euphoria would occur only if drugs bind to the agonist state of the receptor. This provides a simple molecular mechanism to explain opiate antagonist activity. By binding to the receptor in the antagonist state, opiate antagonists reduce the number of receptors that are in the agonist state and are thus capable of mediating morphine effects. Because the extracellular fluid bathing cellular membranes in the brain is rich in sodium, we anticipate that normally the opiate receptor exists predominantly in the sodium, antagonist state. This is consistent with the much greater in vivo potency of antagonists than of agonists. In an environment devoid of sodium, one would predict opiate agonists and antagonists to be equally potent.

The interconversion of the two forms of the opiate receptor presumably involves folding, unfolding, aggregation, disaggregation, or other modifications in protein structure, since the exquisite sensitivity of receptor binding to proteolytic enzymes indicates that the opiate receptor is proteinaceous and contains phospholipid components. Accordingly, one might expect protein-modifying reagents and enzymes that affect protein structure to alter this interconversion.

Since the opiate receptor should normally be largely in the antagonist state, we predict that agents interfering with the interconversion of receptor conformations would selectively reduce agonist binding. Consistent with these predictions is our observation that a variety of protein-modifying reagents and proteolytic enzymes in low concentrations do selectively reduce opiate agonist binding with negligible effects on antagonist binding (Pasternak et al., 1975; Wilson et al., 1975a) (Table 22). Several of these agents, such as N-ethyl-maleimide, iodoacetamide, and mersalyl acid act fairly selectively upon sulfhydryl groups, whereas others, such as N-bromosuccinimide, which primarily affects tryptophan residues, and the proteolytic enzymes trypsin and chymotrypsin, do not act selectively upon sulfhydryl groups. The fact that several different ways of influencing protein structure differentiate agonists and antagonists argues that these agents affect a variety of sites relevant to the interconversion of the two conformations of the opiate receptor. If there were separate agonist and antagonist receptors, as has been suggested by pharmacological evi-

TABLE 22

Differentiation of Receptor Binding of Opiate Agonists and
Antagonists with Protein-Modifying Reagents and Enzymes
[Pert and Snyder, 1974; Wilson et al., 1975a]

Agents	Percent of control	
	Antagonist binding	Agonist binding
Protein-modifying reagents		
N-Ethylmaleimide (0.1 mM)	85	7
Iodoacetamide (5 mM)	90	5
Mersalyl acid (10 μM)	76	23
N-Bromosuccinimide (10 μM)	110	18
Iodine (20 μM)	73	52
2-Methoxy-5-nitrobenzyl bromide (1 mM)	65	50
2-Hydroxy-5-nitrobenzyl bromide (10 mM)	72	47
Enzymes		
Trypsin (1 μg/ml)	65	28
Chymotrypsin (4 μg/ml)	70	15
Phospholipase A (50 ng/ml)	55	15

Antagonist binding utilized 1 nM ^{3}H-naloxone; agonist binding employed 0.6 nM ^{3}H-dihydro-
morphine, both assayed in 100 mM NaCl.

dence, one would have to assume that the agonist receptor possesses
several amino acid residues that are critical for receptor binding and
none of which are components of the antagonist receptor. Perhaps the
agonist receptors are simply more labile to any disruptive influence
than the antagonist receptors. This is unlikely, however, because some
protein-modifying reagents, such as iodine, 2-methoxy-5-nitrobenzyl
bromide, and 2-hydroxy-5-nitrobenzyl bromide, reduce agonist and
antagonist binding to a similar extent.

Other evidence that the effect of the protein-modifying reagents
is related to the sodium-induced interconversion of opiate receptor
conformations derives from the interaction of sodium with protein-
modifying reagents (Pasternak et al., 1975; Wilson et al., 1975a).
Reagents differentiate opiate agonist and antagonist binding best when
incubations are conducted in the presence of sodium. Moreover, the
reagents greatly facilitate the lowering of opiate agonist binding by low
concentrations of sodium. This suggests that these reagents primarily
inhibit the ability of the receptor to assume the agonist or no-sodium
conformation. After treatment with reagents, addition of sodium
transforms the receptor into the sodium state in which it "freezes" so
that it cannot return to the no-sodium state to bind agonists.

140

The postulated interconversion of agonist and antagonist conformations and the influence of sodium resemble models for the behavior of the nicotinic cholinergic receptor (Changeux, 1966; Karlin, 1967; Colquhoun, 1973). In these models, because sodium is the ion whose conductance is altered by nicotinic cholinergic transmission, it is postulated that the binding of sodium to the receptor, in addition to causing a transition between agonist and antagonist conformations, opens the sodium channel, transforming acetylcholine recognition into an excitatory postsynaptic potential. If the endogenous morphine-like substance is a neurotransmitter, one might speculate that sodium is the ion whose conductance is changed by its synaptic activity. The notion that neurotransmitter receptors can exist in separate agonist and antagonist conformations or that the receptors have separate agonist and antagonist sites has been suggested for the receptor for the synaptic activities of glycine, a major inhibitory neurotransmitter in the mammalian central nervous system (Young and Snyder, 1974a,b). Chloride is the ion whose conductance is increased by the inhibitory synaptic activities of glycine. Chloride and other anions inhibit the binding of strychnine, the glycine antagonist, to the glycine receptor in proportion to their ability to mimic the synaptic activites of chloride. Recent evidence suggests that the muscarinic acetylcholine receptor in the brain and guinea pig intestine may exist in distinct agonist and antagonist conformations.* The binding of ^{3}H-quinuclidinyl benzilate (^{3}H-QNB) to the muscarinic receptor is inhibited by muscarinic antagonists in precise proportion to their biological potency in the guinea pig intestine. By contrast, pure muscarinic agonists are up to three orders of magnitude less potent inhibitors of the binding of the antagonist QNB than in eliciting intestinal contractions. Mixed agonist-antagonist muscarinic drugs are intermediate between the actions of agonists and antagonists. This suggests that the muscarinic cholinergic receptor, like the opiate receptor, can exist in two conformations so that pure agonists are relatively weak in binding to the antagonist conformation, which is labeled by ^{3}H-QNB. We speculate that synaptic modulation by interconversion of two receptor forms may be a general property of transmitter receptors, explaining the differential effects of agonists and antagonists and providing a mechanism whereby neurotransmitter recognition can be translated into a change in ion conductance or some other functional property such as cyclic nucleotide formation.

*H.I. Yamamura, K. Chang, and S.H. Snyder, in preparation.

Toward A Concept of Addiction

There are three prominent components of opiate addiction: tolerance, physical dependence, and compulsive craving for opiates. Since craving is difficult to evaluate, we will focus on tolerance and physical dependence. When animals are tolerant to opiates, they require much larger doses of opiate agonists to produce effects formerly elicited with much smaller doses. Thus, tolerance can be looked upon as a state of decreased sensitivity to opiate agonists. Less well known is the fact that as animals become progressively addicted to opiates, they become more sensitive to antagonists. Withdrawal symptoms can be elicited by administering small doses of opiate antagonists to addicted animals, presumably because the antagonists displace the opiate agonists from their receptor sites. Since the bodies of heavily addicted animals contain higher levels of morphine than less addicted animals, one would expect that larger doses of antagonists would be required to precipitate withdrawal in more addicted animals. But the contrary occurs. The dose of naloxone required to precipitate withdrawal symptoms is reduced by as much as two orders of magnitude in severely addicted animals (Way et al., 1969). Thus, addicted animals are *hypersensitive* to opiate antagonists.

This hypersensitivity to antagonists coupled with subsensitivity to agonists in addiction is reminiscent of the properties of the antagonist or sodium form of the opiate receptor as contrasted to the agonist or no-sodium form. We postulate that tolerance and physical dependence to opiates are associated with a change in the opiate receptor so that it is less capable of assuming the agonist form, favoring instead the antagonist, sodium form, much as occurs after treatment with protein-modifying reagents. We have failed to detect systematic alterations in opiate receptor binding in vitro or in vivo that parallel the addictive state. However, it is quite possible that changes in the ability of the receptor to undergo transitions between two states might be lost during the killing and processing of brain tissue for assay. In any event, this concept of addiction provides a working model suggesting numerous experimental approaches.

ABBREVIATIONS

AD_{50}	effective analgesic dose
ADH	antidiuretic hormone
AMPT	α-methylparatyrosine
ARC	Addiction Research Center
ARCI	Addiction Research Center Inventory
ASI	abstinence syndrome intensity
ATP	adenosine triphosphate
cAMP	cyclic adenosine monophosphate
CNS	central nervous system
CTZ	chemoreceptor trigger zone
DA	dopamine
ED_{50}	effective median dose
GABA	γ-aminobutyric acid
5-HT	5-hydroxytryptamine, serotonin
5-HTP	5-hydroxytryptophan
IC_{50}	dose needed to displace binding
MMPI	Minnesota Multiphasic Personality Inventory
NE	norepinephrine
PCPA	p-chlorophenylalanine
PG	prostaglandin
QNB	quinuclidinyl benzilate
TSH	thyroid-stimulating hormone
UTP	uridine triphosphate
VPL	nucleus ventralis posterolateralis
WHO	World Health Organization

BIBLIOGRAPHY

This bibliography contains two types of entries: (1) citations given or work alluded to in the report, and (2) additional references to pertinent literature by conference participants and others. Citations in group (1) may be found in the text on the pages listed in the right-hand column.

Page

Adler, T.K. (1963): The comparative potencies of codeine and its demethylated metabolites after intraventricular injection in the mouse. *J. Pharmacol. Exp. Ther.* 140:155-161.   28,68

Akil, H. and Mayer, D.J. (1972): Antagonism of stimulation-produced analgesia by *p*-CPA, a serotonin synthesis inhibitor. *Brain Res.* 44:692-697.   95

Akil, H., Mayer, D.J., and Liebeskind, J.C. (1972): Comparison chez le rat entre l'analgésie induite par stimulation de la substance grise péri-aqueducale et l'analgésie morphinique. *C. R. Acad. Sci.* 274:3603-3605.   95

Albus, K. (1972): Method for application of drugs into separated parts of the cerebroventricular system. *Physiol. Behav.* 8:569-571.   92

Albus, K. and Herz, A. (1972): Inhibition of behavioural and EEG activation induced by morphine acting on lower brain-stem structures. *Electroencephalogr. Clin. Neurophysiol.* 33:579-590.

Andén, N.-E., Dahlström, A., Fuxe, K., Larsson, K., Olson, L., and Ungerstedt, U. (1966): Ascending monoamine neurons to the telencephalon and diencephalon. *Acta Physiol. Scand.* 67:313-326.   116

Anderson, K.V. and Mahan, P.E. (1971): Increased pain thresholds following combined lesions of thalamic nuclei centrum medianum and centralis lateralis. *Psychon. Sci.* 23:113-114.   91

Andrews, H.L. and Himmelsbach, C.K. (1944): Relation of the intensity of the morphine abstinence syndrome to dosage. *J. Pharmacol. Exp. Ther.* 51:288-293.   124,125

Appelgren, L.-E. and Terenius, L. (1973): Differences in the autoradiographic localization of labelled morphine-like analgesics in the mouse. *Acta Physiol. Scand.* 88:175-182.

Archer, S., Albertson, N.F., Harris, L.S., Pierson, A.K., and Bird, J.G. (1964): Pentazocine. Strong analgesics and analgesic antagonists in the benzomorphan series. *J. Med. Chem.* 7:123-127.   63

Axelrod, J. (1968): Cellular adaptation in the development of tolerance to drugs. *Res. Publ. Assoc. Res. Nerv. Ment. Dis.* 46:247-264.

Banerjee, S.P., Snyder, S.H., Cuatrecasas, P., and Greene, L.A. (1973): Binding of nerve growth factor receptor in sympathetic ganglia. *Proc. Nat. Acad. Sci.* 70:2519-2523.

144

Beaver, W.T., Wallenstein, S.L., Houde, R.W., and Rogers, A. (1969): A comparison   15
of the analgesic effects of profadol and morphine in patients with cancer. *Clin.*
Pharmacol. Ther. 10:314-319.

Bechterew, W.M. (1900): *Les Voies de Conduction du Cerveau et de la Moelle.*   84
Paris: Maloine.

Beecher, H.K. (1946): Pain in men wounded in battle. *Ann. Surg.* 123:96-105.   21

Beecher, H.K. (1959): *Measurement of Subjective Responses: Quantitative Effects*
of Drugs. New York: Oxford University Press.

Beecher, H.K. (1966): Pain: One mystery solved. *Science* 151:840-841.

Belleau, B. (1964): A molecular theory of drug action based on induced   78
conformational perturbations of receptors. *J. Med. Chem.* 7:776-784.

Bennett, V., O'Keefe, E., and Cuatrecasas, P. (1975): Mechanism of action of
cholera toxin and the mobile receptor theory of hormone receptor–adenylate
cyclase interactions. *Proc. Nat. Acad. Sci.* 72:33-37.

Bhargava, H.N., Afifi, A.-H., and Way, E.L. (1973): Effect of chemical sympathec-   112
tomy on morphine antinociception and tolerance development in the rat.
Biochem. Pharmacol. 22:2769-2772.

Bhargava, H.N., Chan, S.L., and Way, E.L. (1975): Influence of hemicholinium   112,116
(HC-3) on morphine analgesia, tolerance, physical dependence and on brain
acetylcholine. *Eur. J. Pharmacol.* (In press)

Bhargava, H.N. and Way, E.L. (1972): Acetylcholinesterase inhibition and   112
morphine effects in morphine tolerant and dependent mice. *J. Pharmacol. Exp.*
Ther. 183:31-40.

Black, M.L. (1963): Sequential blockade as a theoretical basis for drug synergism. *J.*   108
Med. Chem. 6:145-153.

Bläsig, J., Herz, A., and Gramsch, C. (1975): Effects of depletion of brain
catecholamines during the development of morphine dependence on precipitated
withdrawal in rats. *Naunyn-Schmiedebergs Arch. Pharmakol.* (In press)

Bläsig, J., Herz, A., Reinhold, K., and Zieglgänsberger, S. (1973a): Development of
physical dependence on morphine in respect to time and dosage and quantifica-
tion of the precipitated withdrawal syndrome in rats. *Psychopharmacologia*
33:19-38.

Bläsig, J., Reinhold, K., and Herz, A. (1973b): Effect of 6-hydroxydopamine,
5,6-dihydroxytryptamine and raphe lesions on the antinociceptive actions of
morphine in rats. *Psychopharmacologia* 31:111-119.

Bloom, F.E. (1970): Correlating structure and function of synaptic ultrastructure.
In: The Neurosciences: Second Study Program. Schmitt, F.O., editor-in-chief.
New York: Rockefeller University Press, pp. 729-747.

Bloom, F.E. (1972): Amino acids and polypeptides in neuronal function. *Neurosciences Res. Prog. Bull.* 10:122-251. Also *In: Neurosciences Research Symposium Summaries, Vol. 7.* Schmitt, F.O. et al., eds. Cambridge, Mass.: M.I.T. Press, 1974, pp. 122-251.

Bloom, F.E. (1972): Localization of neurotransmitters by electron microscopy. *Res. Publ. Assoc. Res. Nerv. Ment. Dis.* 50:25-57.

Bloom, F.E., Chu, N.-s., Hoffer, B.J., Nelson, C.N., and Siggins, G.R. (1973): Studies on the function of central noradrenergic neurons. *In: Neurosciences Research, Vol. 5. Chemical Approaches to Brain Function.* Ehrenpreis, S. and Kopin, I.J., eds. New York: Academic Press, pp. 54-72.

Bloom, F.E., Iversen, L.L., and Schmitt, F.O. (1970): Macromolecules in synaptic function. *Neurosciences Res. Prog. Bull.* 8:323-455. Also *In: Neurosciences Research Symposium Summaries, Vol. 5.* Schmitt, F.O. et al., eds. Cambridge, Mass.: M.I.T. Press, 1971, pp. 313-439.

Bogoch, A., Roth, J.L.A., and Bockus, H.L. (1954): The effects of morphine on serum amylase and lipase. *Gastroenterology* 26:697-708.   16

Brase, D.A., Tseng, L.F., Loh, H.H., and Way, E.L. (1974): Cholinergic modification of naloxone-induced jumping in morphine-dependent mice. *Eur. J. Pharmacol.* 26:1-8.

Brown, C. (1965): *Manchild in the Promised Land.* New York: Macmillan   13
Publishing Co., Inc.

Bunney, B.S. and Aghajanian, G.K. (1975): Central catecholaminergic neurons: 118
Electrophysiological evidence for pre- and post-synaptic receptors. *In: Pre- and Post-Synaptic Receptors.* Usdin, E. and Bunney, W.E., eds. New York: Marcel Dekker. (In press)

Burnstock, G. (1972): Purinergic nerves. *Pharmacol. Rev.* 24:509-581.   72

Burroughs, W.S. (1962): *Naked Lunch.* New York: Grove Press, Inc.   13

Buxbaum, D.M., Yarbrough, G.G., and Carter, M.E. (1970): Dose-dependent   87
behavioral and analgesic effects produced by microinjection of morphine sulfate (MS) into the anterior thalamic nuclei. *Pharmacologist* 12:211. (Abstr.)

Calesnick, B. and Christensen, J.A. (1967): Latency of cough response as a measure of antitussive agents. *Clin. Pharmacol. Ther.* 8:374-380.

Casey, K.L. and Melzack, R. (1967): Neural mechanisms of pain: a conceptual   22
model. *In: New Concepts in Pain and its Clinical Management.* Way, E.L., ed. Philadelphia: F.A. Davis, pp. 13-31.

Castles, T.R., Campbell, S., Gouge, R., and Lee, C.C. (1972): Nucleic acid synthesis   67
in brains from rats tolerant to morphine analgesia. *J. Pharmacol. Exp. Ther.* 181:399-406.

146

Page

Chakravarty, N.K., Matallana, A., Jensen, R., and Borison, H.L. (1956): Central   16
effects of antitussive drugs on cough and respiration. *J. Pharmacol. Exp. Ther.*
117:127-135.

Chang, H.T. (1973): Integrative action of thalamus in the process of acupuncture   81
for analgesia. *Sci. Sinica* 16:25-60.

Changeux, J.-P. (1966): Responses of acetylcholinesterase from *Torpedo*   140
marmorata to salts and curarizing drugs. *Mol. Pharmacol.* 2:369-392.

Cheney, D.L. and Goldstein, A. (1971): Tolerance to opioid narcotics: Time course
and reversibility of physical dependence in mice. *Nature* 232:477-478.

Clark, W.C. and Yang, J.C. (1974): Acupunctural analgesia? Evaluation by signal   82
detection theory. *Science* 184:1096-1098.

Clark, W.E. LeGros (1932): The structure and connections of the thalamus. *Brain*   84
55:406-470.

Clarke, F.H., Hill, R.T., Saelens, J.K., and Yokoyama, N. (1973): Antagonists in   76
the 5-phenyl-benzomorphan series. *In: Advances in Biochemical Psychopharma-*
cology, Vol. 8. Narcotic Antagonists. Braude, M.C., Harris, L.S., May, E.L.,
Smith, J.P., and Villarreal, J.E., eds. New York: Raven Press, pp. 81-89.

Clouet, D.H., ed. (1971a): *Narcotic Drugs: Biochemical Pharmacology.* New York: 101,104
Plenum Press.

Clouet, D.H. (1971b): Protein and nucleic acid metabolism. *In: Narcotic Drugs:*   102
Biochemical Pharmacology. Clouet, D.H., ed. New York: Plenum Press,
pp. 216-228.

Collier, H.O.J. (1966): Tolerance, physical dependence and receptors. *Adv. Drug*   67
Res. 3:171-188.

Collier, H.O.J. and Roy, A.C. (1974): Morphine-like drugs inhibit the stimulation   43
by E prostaglandins of cyclic AMP formation by rat brain homogenate. *Nature*
248:24-27.

Colquhoun, D. (1973): The relation between classical and cooperative models for   78,140
drug action. *In: Drug Receptors.* Rang, H.P., ed. Baltimore: University Park
Press, pp. 149-182.

Cooper, I.S., Amin, I., Chandra, R., and Waltz, J.M. (1973): A surgical investigation   83
of the clinical physiology of the LP-pulvinar complex in man. *J. Neurol. Sci.*
18:89-110.

Costa, M. and Furness, J.B. (1973): The simultaneous demonstration of adrenergic   110
fibres and enteric ganglion cells. *Histochem. J.* 5:343-349.

Creese, I. and Snyder, S.H. (1975): Receptor binding and pharmacological activity   29,30,31,
in the guinea pig intestine. *J. Pharmacol. Exp. Ther.* (In press)   76

Cuatrecasas, P. (1973a): Cholera toxin-fat cell interaction and the mechanism of   54
activation of the lipolytic response. *Biochemistry* 12:3567-3577.

Cuatrecasas, P. (1973b): Gangliosides and membrane receptors for cholera toxin.   54
Biochemistry 12:3558-3566.

Cuatrecasas, P. (1973c): Insulin receptor of liver and fat cell membranes. *Fed. Proc.*
32:1838-1846.

Cuatrecasas, P. (1973d): The interaction of *Vibrio cholerae* enterotoxin with cell   54
membranes. *Biochemistry* 12:3547-3558.

Cuatrecasas, P. (1973e): *Vibrio cholerae* choleragenoid. Mechanism of inhibition of
cholera toxin action. *Biochemistry* 12:3577-3581.

Cuatrecasas, P. (1974): Insulin receptors, cell membranes and hormone action.
Biochem. Pharmacol. 23:2353-2361.

Cuatrecasas, P. (1974): Membrane receptors. *Annu. Rev. Biochem.* 43:169-214.

Cuello, A.C., Hiley, R., and Iversen, L.L. (1973): Use of catechol *O*-methyl-
transferase for the enzyme radiochemical assay of dopamine. *J. Neurochem.*
21:1337-1340.

Curtis, D.R. and Duggan, A.W. (1969): On the existence of Renshaw cells. *Brain*   80
Res. 15:597-599.

Daniel, E.E., Sutherland, W.H., and Bogoch, A. (1959): Effects of morphine and   16
other drugs on motility of the terminal ileum. *Gastroenterology* 36:510-523.

Deguchi, T. and Axelrod, J. (1973): Supersensitivity and subsensitivity of the
β-adrenergic receptor in pineal gland regulated by catecholamine transmitter.
Proc. Nat. Acad. Sci. 70:2411-2414.

De Meyts, P., Roth, J., Neville, D.M., Jr., Gavin, J.R., III, and Lesniak, M.A.   34
(1973): Insulin interactions with its receptor: Experimental evidence for
negative cooperativity. *Biochem. Biophys. Res. Commun.* 55:154-161.

De Quincey, T. (1822): *Confessions of an English Opium-Eater.* London: Taylor   13
and Hessey.

De Robertis, E. (1971): Molecular biology of synaptic receptors. *Science* 171:   50
963-971.

Dewey, W.L., Snyder, J.W., Harris, L.S., and Howes, J.F. (1969): The effect of
narcotics and narcotic antagonists on the tail-flick response in spinal mice. *J.*
Pharm. Pharmacol. 21:548-550.

Dingledine, R., Goldstein, A., and Kendig, J. (1974): Effects of narcotic opiates   111
and serotonin on the electrical behavior of neurons in the guinea pig myenteric
plexus. *Life Sci.* 14:2299-2309.

Dismukes, K. and Snyder, S.H. (1974): Dynamics of brain histamine. *In: Advances in Neurology, Vol. 5*. New York: Raven Press, pp. 101-109.

Dole, V.P. (1970): Biochemistry of addiction. *Annu. Rev. Biochem.* 39:821-840.

Dole, V.P. (1970): Research on methadone maintenance treatment. *Int. J. Addict.* 5:359-373. Also *In: Methadone Maintenance*. Eisenstein, S., ed. (National

Dole, V.P. (1971): Methadone maintenance treatment for 25,000 heroin addicts. *J. Am. Med. Assoc.* 215:1131-1134.

Dole, V.P. (1972): Detoxification of sick addicts in prison. *J. Am. Med. Assoc.* 220:366-369.

Dole, V.P. (1972): Narcotic addiction, physical dependence and relapse. *N. Engl. J. Med.* 286:988-992.

Dole, V.P. (1973): Heroin addiction—an epidemic disease. *Harvey Lect.* 67:199-211.

Dole, V.P. and Kreek, M.J. (1973): Methadone plasma level: Sustained by a reservoir of drug in tissue. *Proc. Nat. Acad. Sci.* 70:10.

Domino, E.F. (1968): Effects of narcotic analgesics on sensory input, activating system, and motor output. *Res. Publ. Assoc. Res. Nerv. Ment. Dis.* 46:117-149.

Dostrovsky, J. and Pomeranz, B. (1973): Morphine blockade of amino acid putative transmitters on cat spinal cord sensory interneurones. *Nature New Biol.* 246:222-224.   81

Drawbaugh, R. and Lal, H. (1974): Reversal by narcotic antagonist of a narcotic action elicited by a conditional stimulus. *Nature* 247:65-67.

Drew, J.H., Dripps, R.D., and Comroe, J.H. (1946): Clinical studies on morphine. II. The effect of morphine upon the circulation of man and upon the circulatory and respiratory responses to tilting. *Anesthesiology* 7:44-61.   17

Eddy, N.B., Halbach, H., Isbell, H., and Seevers, M.H. (1965): Drug dependence: its significance and characteristics. *Bull. Wld. Hlth. Org.* 32:721-733.   20

Eddy, N.B. and Leimbach, D. (1953): Synthetic analgesics. II. Dithienylbutenyl- and dithienylbutylamines. *J. Pharmacol. Exp. Ther.* 107:385-393.

Eddy, N.B. and May, E.L. (1973): The search for a better analgesic. *Science* 181:407-414.

Eddy, N.B., May, E.L., and Mosettig, E. (1952): Chemistry and pharmacology of the methadols and acetylmethadols. *J. Org. Chem.* 17:321-326.   39

Ehrenpreis, S., Greenberg, J., and Belman, S. (1973): Prostaglandins reverse inhibition of electrically-induced contractions of guinea-pig ileum by morphine, indomethacin and acetylsalicilic acid. *Nature New Biol.* 245:280-282.   43,105

Eidelberg, E. (1975): Acute effects of ethanol and opiates on the nervous system. *In: Research Advances in Alcohol and Drug Problems, Vol. 2.* Gibbons, R., Israel, Y., Kalant, H., Popham, R.E., Schmidt, W., and Smart, R., eds. New York: John Wiley and Sons.

Eidelberg, E. and Barstrow, C.A. (1971): Morphine tolerance and dependence induced by intraventricular injection. *Science* 174:74-76.

Eidelberg, E. and Erspamer, R. (1975): Dopaminergic mechanisms of opiate actions in brain. *J. Pharmacol. Exp. Ther.* 192:50-57.

Eidelberg, E. and Erspamer, R. (1975): Morphine tolerance and dependence are not prevented by an antagonist. *Arch. Int. Pharmacodyn. Ther.* (In press)

Eisenman, A.J.,'Sloan, J.W., Martin, W.R., Jasinski, D.R., and Brooks, J.W. (1969): Catecholamine and 17-hydroxycorticosteroid excretion during a cycle of morphine dependence in man. *J. Psychiatr. Res.* 7:19-28.

El-Mazati, A.M. and Way, E.L. (1971): The biologic disposition of pentazocine in the rat. *J. Pharmacol. Exp. Ther.* 177:332-341.

Emlen, W., Segal, D.S., and Mandell, A.J. (1972): Thyroid state: Effects on pre- and postsynaptic central noradrenergic mechanisms. *Science* 175:79-82.

Fahn, S. and Côte, L.J. (1968): Regional distribution of gamma-aminobutyric acid (GABA) in brain of the rhesus monkey. *J. Neurochem.* 15:209-213.   37

Folch, J., Lees, M., and Sloane-Stanley, G.H. (1957): A simple method for the isolation and purification of total lipids from animal tissues. *J. Biol. Chem.* 226:497-509.   50

Forrest, W.H., Jr. (1970): Report of the Veterans Administration cooperative analgesic study. Presented to the Committee on Problems of Drug Dependence (NAS-NRC). Thirty-Second Meeting, Washington, D.C., 16-18 Feb. 1970.   15

Forrest, W.H., Jr. (1972): Report of the Veterans Administration cooperative analgesic study. Reported to the Committee on Problems of Drug Dependence (NAS-NRC). Thirty-Fourth Annual Scientific Meeting, Ann Arbor, Mich., 22-24 May 1972.   15

Fraser, H.F. and Isbell, H. (1952): Comparative effects of 20 mgm. of morphine sulfate on non-addicts and former morphine addicts. *J. Pharmacol. Exp. Ther.* 105:498-502.   17

Fraser, H.F., Jones, B.E., Rosenberg, D.E., and Thompson, A.K. (1963): Effects of addiction to intravenous heroin on patterns of physical activity in man. *Clin. Pharmacol. Ther.* 4:188-196.   14

Fraser, H.F., Van Horn, G.D., Martin, W.R., Wolbach, A.B., and Isbell, H. (1961): Methods for evaluating addiction liability. (A) "Attitude" of opiate addicts toward opiate-like drugs. (B) A short-term "direct" addiction test. *J. Pharmacol. Exp. Ther.* 133:371-387.   131

150

Frederickson, R.C.A., Horng, J.S., Burgis, V., and Wong, D.T. (1974): Alteration of opiate receptors in physically dependent rats. Reported to the Committee on Problems of Drug Dependence (NAS-NRC). Thirty-Sixth Annual Scientific Meeting, Mexico City, Mexico, 10-14 March 1974.

Friedler, G., Bhargava, H.N., Quock, R., and Way, E.L. (1972): The effect of 6-hydroxydopamine on morphine tolerance and physical dependence. *J. Pharmacol. Exp. Ther.* 183:49-55.   112

Gabella, G. (1972): Fine structure of the myenteric plexus in the guinea-pig ileum. *J. Anat.* 111:69-97.   72

Gates, M. and Montzka, T.A. (1964): Some potent morphine antagonists possessing high analgesic activity. *J. Med. Chem.* 7:127-131.   61

Gershon, M.D. and Altman, R.F. (1971): An analysis of the uptake of 5-hydroxytryptamine by the myenteric plexus of the small intestine of the guinea pig. *J. Pharmacol. Exp. Ther.* 179:29-41.   72

Gintzler, A.R. and Musacchio, J.M. (1974): Interaction between serotonin and morphine in the guinea-pig ileum. *J. Pharmacol. Exp. Ther.* 189:484-492.   108

Goldstein, A. (1973): The search for the opiate receptor. *In: Pharmacology and the Future of Man, Vol. I. Drug Abuse and Contraception.* (Proceedings of the 5th International Congress on Pharmacology, San Francisco, July 1972.) Cochin, J., ed. Basel: S. Karger, pp. 140-150.

Goldstein, A. (1974): Are opiate tolerance and dependence reversible: Implications for the treatment of heroin addiction. *In: Biological and Behavioral Approaches to Drug Dependence.* (Proceedings of the International Symposia on Alcohol and Drug Research, Toronto, October 23-25, 1973.) Cappel H. and LeBlanc, A.E., eds. Toronto, Canada: Addiction Research Foundation.

Goldstein, A. (1974): Opiate receptors. *Life Sci.* 14:615-623.

Goldstein, A., Aronow, L., and Kalman, S.M., eds. (1974): *Principles of Drug Action: The Basis of Pharmacology.* 2nd Ed. New York: John Wiley and Sons.

Goldstein, A., Lowney, L.I., and Pal, B.K. (1971): Stereospecific and nonspecific interactions of the morphine congener levorphanol in subcellular fractions of mouse brain. *Proc. Nat. Acad. Sci.* 68:1742-1747.   25

Goldstein, A. and Schulz, R. (1973): Morphine tolerant-longitudinal muscle strip from guinea-pig ileum. *Br. J. Pharmacol.* 48:655-666.   109

Goldstein, A. and Sheehan, P. (1969): Tolerance to opioid narcotics. I. Tolerance to the "running fit" caused by levorphanol in the mouse. *J. Pharmacol. Exp. Ther.* 169:175-184.

Grumbach, L. and Chernov, H.I. (1965): The analgesic effect of opiate-opiate antagonist combinations in the rat. *J. Pharmacol. Exp. Ther.* 149:385-396.   73

Gyang, E.A. and Kosterlitz, H.W. (1966): Agonist and antagonist actions of morphine-like drugs on the guinea-pig isolated ileum. *Br. J. Pharmacol.* 27:514-527.

16,110

Haertzen, C.A. (1966): Development of scales based on patterns of drug effects, using the Addiction Research Center Inventory (ARCI). *Psychol. Rep.* 18:163-194.

13,14, 133

Hardy, R.A., Jr. and Howell, M.G. (1965): Synthetic analgetics with morphine-like actions. *In: Analgetics.* deStevens, G., ed. New York: Academic Press, pp. 179-279.

39

Henderson, G., Hughes, J., and Kosterlitz, H.W. (1972): A new example of a morphine-sensitive neuro-effector junction: Adrenergic transmission in the mouse vas deferens. *Br. J. Pharmacol.* 46:764-766.

Henderson, G., Hughes, J., and Thompson, J.W. (1972): The variation of noradrenaline output with frequency of nerve stimulation and the effect of morphine on the cat nictitating membrane and on the guinea-pig myenteric plexus. *Br. J. Pharmacol.* 46:524P-525P.

Herz, A. (1973): Central nervous sites of action of morphine in dependent and nondependent rabbits. *In: Pharmacology and the Future of Man, Vol. 1. Drug Abuse and Contraception.* (Proceedings of the 5th International Congress on Pharmacology, San Francisco, July 1972.) Cochin, J., ed. Basel: S. Karger, pp. 125-139.

Herz, A., Albus, K., Metyš, J., Schubert, P., and Teschemacher, Hj. (1970): On the central sites for the antinociceptive action of morphine and fentanyl. *Neuropharmacology* 9:539-551.

87

Herz, A. and Bläsig, J. (1974): Neurobiologische Aspekte der Morphin-Abhängigkeit. *Naturwissenschaften* 61:232-238.

Herz, A., Bläsig, J., and Papeschi, R. (1974): Role of catecholaminergic mechanisms in the expression of the morphine abstinence syndrome in rats. *Psychopharmacologia* 39:121-143.

Herz, A. and Reinhold, K. (1973): Modification of precipitated withdrawal in the rat by influencing catecholaminergic mechanisms acutely and chronically. *Naunyn-Schmiedebergs Arch. Pharmakol.* 277(Suppl.):R30. (Abstr.)

Herz, A. and Teschemacher, Hj. (1971): Activities and sites of antinociceptive actions of morphine-like analgesics. *Adv. Drug Res.* 6:79-119.

27

Herz, A. and Teschemacher, Hj. (1973): Development of tolerance to the antinociceptive effect of morphine after intraventricular injection. *Experientia* 29:64-65.

Herz, A., Teschemacher, Hj., Albus, K., and Zieglgänsberger, S. (1972): Morphine abstinence syndrome in rabbits precipitated by injection of morphine antagonists into the ventricular system and restricted parts of it. *Psychopharmacologia* 26:219-235.

92

Hiller, J.M., Pearson, J., and Simon, E.J. (1973): Distribution of stereospecific   35,43,44,
binding of the potent narcotic analgesic etorphine in the human brain: 89
Predominance in the limbic system. *Res. Commun. Chem. Pathol. Pharmacol.*
6:1052-1062.

Hiller, J.M. and Simon E.J. (1973): Inhibition by levorphanol of the induction of
acetylcholinesterase in a mouse neuroblastoma cell line. *J. Neurochem.*
20:1789-1792.

Himmelsbach, C.K. (1941): The morphine abstinence syndrome, its nature and   124
treatment. *Ann. Int. Med.* 15:829-839.

Hitzemann, R.J., Hitzemann, B.A., and Loh, H.H. (1974): Binding of ^{3}H-naloxone
in the mouse brain: Effect of ions and tolerance development. *Life Sci.*
14:2393-2404.

Hitzemann, R.J. and Loh, H.H. (1973): Characteristics of the binding of   27
^{3}H-naloxone in the mouse brain. *In: Program and Abstracts, Society for
Neuroscience.* Third Annual Meeting, San Diego, Calif., p. 350.

Ho, I.K., Brase, D.A., Loh, H.H., and Way, E.L. (1975): Influence of L-tryptophan   114
on morphine analgesia, tolerance and physical dependence. *J. Pharmacol. Exp.
Ther.* (In press)

Ho, I.K., Loh, H.H., and Way, E.L. (1972a): Effect of cyclic AMP on morphine
analgesia tolerance and physical dependence. *Nature* 238:397-398.

Ho, I.K., Loh, H.H., and Way, E.L. (1972b): Effect of l-tryptophan on morphine   112
analgesia, tolerance and physical dependence. Reported to the Committee on
Problems of Drug Dependence (NAS-NRC). Thirty-Fourth Annual Scientific
Meeting, Ann Arbor, Mich., 22-24 May 1972.

Ho, I.K., Loh, H.H., and Way, E.L. (1972c): Mini thin-layer chromatography in the
detection of narcotics in urine from subjects on a methadone maintenance
program. *J. Chromatogr.* 65:577-579.

Ho, I.K., Loh, H.H., and Way, E.L. (1973a): Cyclic adenosine monophosphate   113
antagonism of morphine analgesia. *J. Pharmacol. Exp. Ther.* 185:336-346.

Ho, I.K., Loh, H.H., and Way, E.L. (1973b): Effects of cyclic 3',5'-adenosine   113,114
monophosphate on morphine tolerance and physical dependence. *J. Pharmacol.
Exp. Ther.* 185:347-357.

Ho, I.K., Loh, H.H., and Way, E.L. (1973c): Influence of 5,6-dihydroxytryptamine   112,113
on morphine tolerance and physical dependence. *Eur. J. Pharmacol.* 21:331-336.

Ho, I.K., Lu, S.E., Stolman, S., Loh, H.H., and Way, E.L. (1972d): Influence of
p-chlorphenylalanine on morphine tolerance and physical dependence and
regional brain serotonin turnover studies in morphine tolerant-dependent mice.
J. Pharmacol. Exp. Ther. 182:155-165.

Hollenberg, M.D. and Cuatrecasas, P., (1973): Epidermal growth factor: Receptors in human fibroblasts and modulation of action by cholera toxin. *Proc. Nat. Acad. Sci.* 70:2964-2968.

Hollenberg, M.D., Fishman, P.H., Bennett, V., and Cuatrecasas, P. (1974): Cholera toxin and cell growth: Role of membrane gangliosides. *Proc. Nat. Acad. Sci.* 71:4224-4228.

Hopton, D.S. and Torrance, H.B. (1967): Action of various new analgesic drugs on human common bile duct. *Gut* 8:296-300.   16

Houde, R.W., Wallenstein, S.L., and Rogers, A. (1970): Clinical analgesic assays: Progress report from Sloan-Kettering Institute for Cancer Research. Reported to the Committee on Problems of Drug Dependence (NAS-NRC). Thirty-Second Meeting, Washington, D.C., 16-18 Feb. 1970.   15

Houde, R.W., Wallenstein, S.L., and Rogers, A. (1972): Analgesic studies program of the Sloan-Kettering Institute for Cancer Research. Reported to the Committee on Problems of Drug Dependence (NAS-NRC). Thirty-Fourth Annual Scientific Meeting, Ann Arbor, Mich., 22-24 May 1972.   15

Hughes, J. (1973): Differential labelling of intraneuronal noradrenaline stores with different concentrations of (−)-3H-noradrenaline. *Br. J. Pharmacol.* 47:428-430.

Hughes, J., Kosterlitz, H.W., and Leslie, F.M. (1974): Assessment of the agonist and antagonist activities of narcotic analgesic drugs by means of the mouse vas deferens. *Br. J. Pharmacol.* 51:139P-140P.   70

Iggo, A. (1959): Cutaneous heat and cold receptors with slowly conducting (C) afferent fibres. *Q. J. Exp. Physiol.* 44:362-370.   21

Ingoglia, N.A. and Dole, V.P. (1970): Localization of *d*- and *l*-methadone after intraventricular injection into rat brains. *J. Pharmacol. Exp. Ther.* 175:84-87.

Irwin, S., Houde, R.W., Bennett, D.R., Hendershot, L.C., and Seevers, M.H. (1951): The effects of morphine, methadone and meperidine on some reflex responses of spinal animals to nociceptive stimulation. *J. Pharmacol. Exp. Ther.* 101:132-143.

Isbell, H. and Chruściel, T.L. (1970): Dependence liability of "non-narcotic" drugs. *Bull. Wld. Hlth. Org.* 43(Suppl.):1-111.   19,20

Iversen, L.L. (1973): Catecholamine uptake processes. *Br. Med. Bull.* 29:130-135.

Iversen, L.L., Kelly, J.S., Minchin, M., Schon, F., and Snodgrass, S.R. (1973): Role of amino acids and peptides in synaptic transmission. *Brain Res.* 62:567-576.

Iwamoto, E.T. (1974): Circling behavior precipitated by naloxone in morphine dependent rats with unilateral lesions of the substantia nigra. *Fed. Proc.* 33:487. (Abstr.)

154

Iwamoto, E.T., Ho, I.K., and Way, E.L. (1973): Elevation of brain dopamine during   115,116
naloxone-precipitated withdrawal in morphine-dependent mice and rats. *J.*
Pharmacol. Exp. Ther. 187:558-567.

Jacobowitz, D. (1965): Histochemical studies of the autonomic innervation of the   110
gut. *J. Pharmacol. Exp. Ther.* 149:358-364.

Jacobson, A.E. (1972): Narcotic analgesics and antagonists. *In: Chemical and*
Biological Aspects of Drug Dependence. Mulé, S.J. and Brill, H., eds. Cleveland,
Ohio: Chemical Rubber Co. Press, pp. 101-118.

Jacobson, A.E. (1975): Hansch analysis of the 6,7-benzomorphan analgesics. *J.*   64
Med. Chem. (In press)

Jacquet, Y.F. and Lajtha, A. (1973): Morphine action at central nervous sites in   87
rat: Analgesia or hyperalgesia depending on site and dose. *Science* 182:490-492.

Jaffe, J.H. (1966): Narcotic analgesics. *In: The Pharmacological Basis for*
Therapeutics. Goodman, L.S. and Gilman, A., eds. New York: Macmillan Co.,
pp. 247-284.

Jasinski, D.R. and Mansky, P.A. (1970): The subjective effects of GPA 2087 and   15
nalbuphine (EN-2234A). Reported to the Committee on Problems of Drug
Dependence (NAS-NRC). Thirty-Fourth Annual Scientific Meeting, Washington,
D.C., 16-18 Feb. 1970.

Jasinski, D.R. and Mansky, P.A. (1972): Evaluation of nalbuphine for abuse   15
potential. *Clin. Pharmacol. Ther.* 13:78-90.

Jasinski, D.R., Martin, W.R., and Haertzen, C.A. (1967): The human pharmacology   126
and abuse potential of N-allylnoroxymorphone (naloxone). *J. Pharmacol. Exp.*
Ther. 157:420-426.

Jasinski, D.R., Martin, W.R., and Hoeldtke, R.D. (1970): Effects of short- and   61
long-term administration of pentazocine in man. *Clin. Pharmacol. Ther.*
11:385-403.

Jasinski, D.R., Martin, W.R., and Hoeldtke, R. (1971): Studies of the dependence-   59,125
producing properties of GPA-1657, profadol, and propiram in man. *Clin.*
Pharmacol. Ther. 12:613-649.

Jasinski, D.R., Martin, W.R., and Sapira, J.D. (1968): Antagonism of the subjective,
behavioral, pupillary, and respiratory depressant effects of cyclazocine by
naloxone. *Clin. Pharmacol. Ther.* 9:215-222.

Jongh, D.K. de and van Proosdij-Hartzema, E.G. (1957): Pharmacology of (±)-, (+)-   39
and (−)-2:2-diphenyl-3-methyl-4-morpholino-butyryl-pyrrolidine. *J. Pharm.*
Pharmacol. 9:730-738.

Jurna, I., Grossmann, W., and Theres, C. (1973): Inhibition by morphine of   81
repetitive activation of cat spinal motoneurones. *Neuropharmacology*
12:983-993.

Kaelber, W.W. and Mitchell, C.L. (1967): The centrum medianum-central tegmental   91
fasciculus complex. A stimulation, lesion and degeneration study in the cat.
Brain 90:83-100.

Karlin, A. (1967): On the application of "a plausible model" of allosteric proteins   78,140
to the receptor for acetylcholine. *J. Theor. Biol.* 16:306-320.

Kay, D.C., Eisenstein, R.B., and Jasinski, D.R. (1969): Morphine effects on human   14
REM state, waking state and NREM sleep. *Psychopharmacologia* 14:404-416.

Klee, W.A. and Streaty, R.A. (1974): Narcotic receptor sites in morphine-   27
dependent rats. *Nature* 248:61-63.

Klotz, I.M. (1950): The nature of some ion-protein complexes. *Cold Spring Harbor*   46
Symp. Quant. Biol. 14:97-112.

Knapp, S. and Mandell, A.J. (1972): Narcotic drugs: Effects on the serotonin   104
biosynthetic systems of the brain. *Science* 177:1209-1211.

Knapp, S. and Mandell, A.J. (1973): Short- and long-term lithium administration:
Effects on the brain's serotonergic biosynthetic systems. *Science* 180:645-647.

Kolb, L. (1925): Pleasure and deterioration from narcotic addiction. *Ment. Hyg.*   14
9:699-724.

Korf, J., Bunney, B.S., and Aghajanian, G.K. (1974): Noradrenergic neurons: 81
Morphine inhibition of spontaneous activity. *Eur. J. Pharmacol.* 25:165-169.

Kosterlitz, H.W., Lord, J.A.H., and Watt, A.J. (1973a): Morphine receptor in the   64,68,69,
myenteric plexus of the guinea-pig ileum. *In: Agonist and Antagonist Actions of*   70
Narcotic Analgesic Drugs. Kosterlitz, H.W., Collier, H.O.J., and Villarreal, J.E.,
eds. Baltimore: University Park Press, pp. 45-61.

Kosterlitz, H.W. and Lydon, R.J. (1971): Impulse transmission in the myenteric
plexus-longitudinal muscle preparation of the guinea-pig ileum. *Br. J. Pharmacol.*
43:74-85.

Kosterlitz, H.W. and Waterfield, A.A. (1975): In vitro models in the study of   29,64,68,
structure-activity relationships of narcotic analgesics. *Annu. Rev. Pharmacol.* (In   69,70
press)

Kosterlitz, H.W., Waterfield, A.A. and Berthoud, V. (1973b): Assessment of the   29,64,68,
agonist and antagonist properties of narcotic analgesic drugs by their actions on   69,70,71
the morphine receptor in the guinea pig ileum. *In: Advances in Biochemical*
Psychopharmacology, Vol. 8. Narcotic Antagonists. Braude, M.C., Harris, L.S.,
May, E.L., Smith, J.P., and Villarreal, J.E., eds. New York: Raven Press,
pp. 319-334.

Kosterlitz, H.W. and Watt, A.J. (1968): Kinetic parameters of narcotic agonists and   41,69,70
antagonists, with particular reference to *N*-allylnoroxymorphone (naloxone). *Br.*
J. Pharmacol. 33:266-276.

Krantz, J.C., Eddy, N.B., Jacobson, A.E., and Kaufman, J.J. (1971): Narcotic agonists and antagonists. *CMD Selected Speeches*, pp. 329-342.

Krueger, H., Eddy, N.B., and Sumwalt, M. (1941): *The Pharmacology of Opium Alkaloids. Publ. Hlth. Rep.* Suppl. 165. (U.S. Government Printing Office)   13

Kuczenski, R.T. and Mandell, A.J. (1972): Allosteric activation of hypothalamic tyrosine hydroxylase by ions and sulphated mucopolysaccharides. *J. Neurochem.* 19:131-137.

Kudo, T., Yoshii, N., Shimizu, S., Aikawa, S., and Nakahama, H. (1966): Effects of   83
stereotaxic thalamotomy to intractable pain and numbness. *Keio J. Med.* 15:191-194.

Kudo, T., Yoshii, N., Shimizu, S., Aikawa, S., Nishioka, S., and Nakahama, H.   83
(1968): Stereotaxic thalamotomy for pain relief. *Tohoku J. Exp. Med.* 96:219-234.

Kuhar, M.J., Pert, C.B., and Snyder, S.H. (1973): Regional distribution of opiate   35,36,37,
receptor binding in monkey and human brain. *Nature* 245:447-450.   43,53,89

Lasagna, L., von Felsinger, J.M., and Beecher, H.K. (1955): Drug-induced mood   15
changes in man. I. Observations on healthy subjects, chronically ill patients, and "postaddicts." *J. Am. Med. Assoc.* 157:1006-1020.

Laschka, E., Teschemacher, Hj., Mehraein, D., and Herz, A. (1974): Site of action   92
of morphine in the development of physical dependence in rats. *Naunyn-Schmiedebergs Arch. Pharmakol.* 282(Suppl.): R54. (Abstr.)

Lee, C.Y., Stolman, S., Akera, T., and Brody, T.M. (1973): Saturable binding of   27
[^{3}H]dihydromorphine to rat brain tissue *in vitro:* characterization and effect of morphine pretreatment. *Pharmacologist* 15:202. (Abstr.)

Lees, G.M., Kosterlitz, H.W., and Waterfield, A.A. (1973): Characteristics of morphine-sensitive release of neuro-transmitter substances. *In: Agonist and Antagonist Actions of Narcotic Analgesic Drugs.* Kosterlitz, H.W., Collier, H.O.J., and Villarreal, J.E., eds. Baltimore: University Park Press, pp 142-152.

Liebeskind, J.C., Guilbaud, G., Besson, J.-M., and Oliveras, J.-L. (1973): Analgesia   91,94
from electrical stimulation of the periaqueductal gray matter in the cat: behavioral observations and inhibitory effects on spinal cord interneurons. *Brain Res.* 50:441-446.

Liebeskind, J.C. and Mayer, D.J. (1971): Somatosensory evoked responses in the   97
mesencephalic central gray matter of the rat. *Brain Res.* 27:133-151.

Liebeskind, J.C., Mayer, D.J., and Akil, H. (1974): Central mechanisms of pain inhibition: Studies of analgesia from focal brain stimulation. *In: Advances in Neurology, Vol. 4. International Symposium on Pain.* Bonica, J.J., ed. New York: Raven Press, pp. 261-268.

Liebman, J.M., Mayer, D.J., and Liebeskind, J.C. (1973): Self-stimulation loci in the midbrain central gray matter of the rat. *Behav. Biol.* 9:299-306.

Lindvall, O., Björklund, A., Nobin, A., and Stenevi, U. (1974): The adrenergic innervation of the rat thalamus as revealed by the glyoxylic acid fluorescence method. *J. Comp. Neurol.* 154:317-348.   87

Loh, H.H., Cho, T.M., Wu, Y.-C., and Way, E.L. (1974): Stereospecific binding of narcotics to brain cerebrosides. *Life Sci.* 14:2231-2245.

Loh, H.H., Hitzemann, R.J., and Way, E.L. (1973): Effect of acute morphine administration on the metabolism of brain catecholamines. *Life Sci.* 12:33-41.

Loh, H.H., Shen, F.-H., and Way, E.L. (1969): Inhibition of morphine tolerance and physical dependence development and brain serotonin synthesis by cycloheximide. *Biochem. Pharmacol.* 18:2711-2721.   103

Loh, H.H., Shen, F.-H., and Way, E.L. (1971): Effect of dactinomycin on the acute toxicity and brain uptake of morphine. *J. Pharmacol. Exp. Ther.* 177:326-331.

Lomax, P. and George, R. (1966): Thyroid activity following administration of morphine in rats with hypothalamic lesions. *Brain Res.* 2:361-367.   17

Lowney, L.I., Schulz, K., Lowery, P.J., and Goldstein, A. (1974): Partial purification of an opiate receptor from mouse brain. *Science* 183:749-753.

McClane, T.K. and Martin, W.R. (1967a): Antagonism of the spinal cord effects of morphine and cyclazocine by naloxone and thebaine. *Int. J. Neuropharmacol.* 6:325-327.   80

McClane, T.K. and Martin, W.R. (1967b): Effects of morphine, nalorphine, cyclazocine, and naloxone on the flexor reflex. *Int. J. Neuropharmacol.* 6:89-98.   80

Mandell, A.J. (1973): Neurobiological barriers to euphoria. *Am. Sci.* 61:565-573.

Mandell, A.J. (1973): Redundant macromolecular mechanisms in central synaptic regulation. *In: New Concepts in Neurotransmitter Regulation.* Mandell, A.J., ed. New York: Plenum Press, pp. 259-277.

Mandell, A.J. and Karno, M. (1972): Isolation and neurochemical sensitization—A counterintuitive hypothesis. *In: Research and Relevance, Vol. 21. Science and Psychoanalysis.* Masserman, J.H., ed. New York: Grune and Stratton, pp. 13-29.

Mandell, A.J., Knapp, S., Kuczenski, R.T., and Segal, D.S. (1972): Methamphetamine-induced alteration in the physical state of rat caudate tyrosine hydroxylase. *Biochem. Pharmacol.* 21:2737-2750.

Mandell, A.J., Segal, D.S., and Kuczenski, R. (1974): Metabolic adaptation to antidepressant drugs—A neurochemical paradox. *In: Catecholamines and Behavior.* Friedhoff, A.J., ed. New York: Plenum Press. (In press)

158

Mandell, A.J., Segal, D.S., Kuczenski, R.T., and Knapp, S. (1972): Some macromolecular mechanisms in CNS neurotransmitter pharmacology and their psychobiological organization. *In: The Chemistry of Mood, Motivation, and Memory*. McGaugh, J.L., ed. New York: Plenum Press, pp. 105-148.

Mandell, A.J., Segal, D.S., Kuczenski, R.T., and Knapp, S. (1973): Amphetamine-induced changes in the regulation of neurotransmitter biosynthetic and receptor functions in the brain. *In: Pharmacology and the Future of Man, Vol. I. Drug Abuse and Contraception*. (Proceedings of the 5th International Congress on Pharmacology, San Francisco, July 1972.) Cochin, J. ed. Basel: S. Karger, pp. 95-105.

Mark, V.H. and Ervin, F.R. (1969): Stereotactic surgery for the relief of pain. *In: Pain and the Neurosurgeon. A Forty-Year Experience*. White, J.C. and Sweet, W.H. Springfield, Ill.: C.C Thomas.   83

Martin, W.R. (1966): Assessment of the dependence producing potentiality of narcotic analgesics. *In: International Encyclopedia of Pharmacology and Therapeutics, Sec. 6, Vol. 1. Clinical Pharmacology*. Lasagna, L., ed. Glasgow, Scotland: Pergamon Press, pp. 155-180.   126,131

Martin, W.R. (1967): Opioid antagonists. *Pharmacol. Rev.* 19:463-521.

Martin, W.R. (1968): A homeostatic and redundancy theory of tolerance to and dependence on narcotic analgesics. *Res. Publ. Assoc. Res. Nerv. Ment. Dis.* 46:206-223.

Martin, W.R. (1970): Pharmacological redundancy as an adaptive mechanism in the central nervous system. *Fed. Proc.* 29:13-18.   127

Martin, W.R. and Eades, C.G. (1961): Demonstration of tolerance and physical dependence in the dog following a short-term infusion of morphine. *J. Pharmacol. Exp. Ther.* 133:262-270.

Martin, W.R., Eades, C.G., Thompson, W.O., Thompson, J.A., and Flanary, H.G. (1974): Morphine physical dependence in the dog. *J. Pharmacol. Exp. Ther.* 189:759-771.

Martin, W.R., Fraser, H.F., Gorodetzky, C.W., and Rosenberg, D.E. (1965): Studies of the dependence-producing potential of the narcotic antagonist 2-cyclopropyl-methyl-2'-hydroxy-5,9-dimethy-6,7-benzomorphan (cyclazocine, Win-20, 740, ARC II-C-3). *J. Pharmacol. Exp. Ther.* 150:426-436.   130

Martin, W.R. and Gorodetzky, C.W. (1965): Demonstration of tolerance to and physical dependence on N-allylnormorphine (nalorphine). *J. Pharmacol. Exp. Ther.* 150:437-442.   130

Martin, W.R., Gorodetzky, C.W., and McClane, T.K. (1966): An experimental study in the treatment of narcotic addicts with cyclazocine. *Clin. Pharmacol. Ther.* 7:455-465.   18,19,61

Martin, W.R., Gorodetzky, C.W., and Thompson, W.O. (1973a): Receptor dualism: some kinetic implications. *In: Agonist and Antagonist Actions of Narcotic Analgesic Drugs.* Kosterlitz, H.W., Collier, H.O.J., and Villarreal, J.E., eds. Baltimore: University Park Press, pp. 30-44.

Martin, W.R. and Jasinski, D.R. (1969): Physiological parameters of morphine dependence in man—tolerance, early abstinence, protracted abstinence. *J. Psychiatr. Res.* 7:9-17.   126,127, 129

Martin, W.R. and Jasinski, D.R. (1972): The mode of action and abuse potentiality of narcotic antagonists. *In: Pain, Basic Principles—Pharmacology—Therapy.* Janzen, R., Keidel, W.D., Herz, A., and Steichele, C., eds. Stuttgart: Georg Thieme Publishers; English Ed., Payne, J.P. and Burt, R.A.P., eds. London: Churchill Livingstone, pp. 225-234.

Martin, W.R., Jasinski, D.R., Haertzen, C.A., Kay, D.C., Jones, B.E., Mansky, P.A., and Carpenter, R.W. (1973b): Methadone—a re-evaluation. *Arch. Gen. Psychiatry* 28:286-295.   131,132, 133,134

Martin, W.R., Jasinski, D.R., and Mansky, P.A. (1973c): Naltrexone, an antagonist for the treatment of heroin dependence. *Arch. Gen. Psychiatry* 28:784-791.   61

Martin, W.R., Jasinski, D.R., Sapira, J.D., Flanary, H.G., Kelly, O.A., Thompson, A.K., and Logan, C.R. (1968): The respiratory effects of morphine during a cycle of dependence. *J. Pharmacol. Exp. Ther.* 162:182-189.   127,128, 129

May, E.L. (1974): Research toward non-abusive analgesics. *In: Psychopharmacological Agents, Vol. III.* Gordon, M., ed. New York: Academic Press. (In press)

Mayer, D. and Hayes, R. (1974): Narcotic and stimulation-produced analgesia: Tolerance and cross-tolerance. *Fed. Proc.* 33:502. (Abstr.)

Mayer, D.J., and Liebeskind, J.C. (1974): Pain reduction by focal electrical stimulation of the brain: An anatomical and behavioral analysis. *Brain Res.* 68:73-93.   94,95,97

Mayer, D.J., Wolfle, T.L., Akil, H., Carder, B., and Liebeskind, J.C. (1971): Analgesia from electrical stimulation in the brainstem of the rat. *Science* 174:1351-1354.   91,94

Mehler, W.R., Feferman, M.E., and Nauta, W.J.H. (1960): Ascending axon degeneration following anterolateral cordatomy. An experimental study in the monkey. *Brain* 83:718-750.   84,91

Melzack, R. (1973): *The Puzzle of Pain.* Middlesex, England: Penguin Books Ltd.   86

Melzack, R., Stotler, W.A., and Livingston, W.K. (1958): Effects of discrete brainstem lesions in cats on perception of noxious stimulation. *J. Neurophysiol.* 21:353-367.   91

Melzack, R. and Wall, P.D. (1965): Pain mechanisms: A new theory. *Science* 150:971-979.   21

160

Page

Mitchell, C.L. and Kaelber, W.W. (1966): Effect of medial thalamic lesions on responses elicited by tooth pulp stimulation. *Am. J. Physiol.* 210:263-269.   91

Mokrasch, L.C. (1967): A rapid purification of proteolipid protein adaptable to large quantities. *Life Sci.* 6:1905-1909.   50

Monod, J., Wyman, J., and Changeux, J.-P. (1965): On the nature of allosteric transitions: a plausible model. *J. Mol. Biol.* 12:88-118.   78

Moricca, G. (1974): Chemical hypophysectomy for cancer pain. *Adv. Neurol.* 4:707-714.   83

Mulder, A.H., Yamamura, H.I., Kuhar, M.J., and Snyder, S.H. (1974): Release of acetylcholine from hippocampal slices by potassium depolarization: dependence on high affinity choline uptake. *Brain Res.* 70:372-376.

Nashold, B.S., Wilson, W.P., and Slaughter, D.G. (1969): Sensations evoked by stimulation in the midbrain of man. *J. Neurosurg.* 30:14-24.   91

Nauta, W.J.H. (1958): Hippocampal projections and related neural pathways to the midbrain in the cat. *Brain* 81:319-340.   86

Nomof, N., Elliott, H.W., and Parker, K. (1968): Reported to the Committee on Problems of Drug Dependence (NAS-NRC). Thirtieth Meeting, 1968.   15

North, R.B., Harik, S.I., and Snyder, S.H. (1974): Amphetamine isomers: Influences on locomotor and stereotyped behavior of cats. *Pharmacol. Biochem. Behav.* 2:115-118.

Olds, M.E. and Olds, J. (1963): Approach-avoidance analysis of rat diencephalon. *J. Comp. Neurol.* 120:259-295.   91

Papeschi, R., Theiss, P., and Herz, A. (1974): Serotonin and dopamine turnover after acute and chronic morphine administration. *Arzneimittel-Forsch. (Drug Res.)* 24:1017-1019.

Pasternak, G.W. and Snyder, S.H. (1974): Opiate receptor binding: Effects of enzymatic treatments. *Mol. Pharmacol.* 10:183-193.   43,54,76

Pasternak, G.W. and Snyder, S.H. (1975): Identification of novel high affinity opiate receptor binding in rat brain. *Nature* 253:563-565.   31,32,33, 34,50,54

Pasternak, G.W., Wilson, H.A., and Snyder, S.H. (1975): Differential effects of protein modifying reagents on receptor binding of opiate agonists and antagonists. *Mol. Pharmacol.* (In press)   34,54,137, 138,139

Paton, W.D.M. (1957): The action of morphine and related substances on contraction and on acetylcholine output of coaxially stimulated guinea-pig ileum. *Br. J. Pharmacol. Chemother.* 12:119-127.   16

Perl, E.R. (1972): Mode of action of nociceptors. *In: Cervical Pain.* Hirsch, C. and Zotterman, Y., eds. New York: Pergamon Press, pp. 157-164.   21

Pert, A. and Yaksh, T.L. (1974a): The neuroanatomical and neurochemical 88
substrates underlying morphine induced analgesia in the rhesus monkey.
Reported to the Committee on Problems of Drug Dependence (NAS-NRC).
Thirty-Sixth Annual Scientific Meeting, Mexico City, Mexico, 10-14 March
1974.

Pert, A. and Yaksh, T. (1974b): Sites of morphine induced analgesia in the primate 88,90
brain: relation to pain pathways. *Brain Res.* 80:135-140.

Pert, A. and Yaksh, T. (1975): Localization of the antinociceptive action of 88
morphine in primate brain. *Physiol. Behav.* (In press)

Pert, C.B. (1974): The opiate receptor: Its demonstration, properties and 26
distribution. Doctoral Dissertation, The Johns Hopkins University, Baltimore,
Maryland.

Pert, C.B., Aposhian, D., and Snyder, S.H. (1974a): Phylogenetic distribution of
opiate receptor binding. *Brain Res.* 75:356-361.

Pert, C.B., Pasternak, G., and Snyder, S.H. (1973): Opiate agonists and antagonists 44,67,74
discriminated by receptor binding in brain. *Science* 182:1359-1361.

Pert, C.B., Snowman, A.M., and Snyder, S.H. (1974b): Localization of opiate 38
receptor binding in synaptic membranes of rat brain. *Brain Res.* 70:184-188.

Pert, C.B. and Snyder, S.H. (1973a): Opiate receptor: Demonstration in nervous 26,29,44,
tissue. *Science* 179:1011-1014. 74

Pert, C.B. and Snyder, S.H. (1973b): Properties of opiate-receptor binding in rat 28,31,33,
brain. *Proc. Nat. Acad. Sci.* 70:2243-2247. 69,74

Pert, C.B. and Snyder, S.H. (1974): Opiate receptor binding of agonists and 54,64,74,
antagonists affected differentially by sodium. *Mol. Pharmacol.* 10:868-879. 75,76,77,
137,139

Pert, C.B., Snyder, S.H., and May, E.L. (1975): Opiate receptor interaction of 74,75,77
benzomorphans in rat brain homogenates. *J. Pharmacol. Exp. Ther.* (In press)

Pierson, A.K. (1973): Assays for narcotic antagonist activity in rodents. *In:* 74
Advances in Biochemical Psychopharmacology, Vol. 8. Narcotic Antagonists.
Braude, M.C., Harris, L.S., May, E.L., Smith, J.P., and Villarreal, J.E., eds. New
York: Raven Press, pp. 245-261.

Pohl, J. (1915): Ueber das N-Allylnorcodein, einen Antagonisten des Morphins. *Z.* 61
Exp. Pathol. Ther. 17:370-382.

Pomeranz, B. (1973): Specific nociceptive fibers projecting from spinal cord
neurons to the brain: a possible pathway for pain. *Brain Res.* 50:447-451.

Reinhold, K., Bläsig, J., and Herz, A. (1973): Changes in brain concentration of
biogenic amines and the antinociceptive effect of morphine in rats. *Naunyn-
Schmiedebergs Arch. Pharmakol.* 278:69-80.

162

Reynolds, A.K. and Randall, L.O. (1957): *Morphine and Allied Drugs.* Toronto: 13
University of Toronto Press.

Richardson, D.E. and Akil, H. (1973): Acute relief of intractable pain by brain
stimulation in human patients. Paper presented at Annual Meeting of American
Association of Neurological Surgeons, 1973.

Richardson, D.E. and Akil, H. (1974): Chronic relief of intractable pain by brain   95,99
stimulation in human patients. Paper presented at the Society for Neurological
Surgery Meeting, St. Louis, April, 1974.

Richardson, D.E. and Zorub, D.S. (1970): Sensory function of the pulvinar.   83
Confin. Neurol. 32:165-173.

Robinson, R.G. and Gershon, M.D. (1971): Synthesis and uptake of 5-hydroxy-   109
tryptamine by the myenteric plexus of the guinea pig ileum: a histochemical
study. *J. Pharmacol. Exp. Ther.* 178:311-324.

Ross, L.L. and Gershon, M.D. (1972): Electron microscopic radioautographic and   109
fluorescence localization of the sites of 5-hydroxytryptamine (5-HT) uptake in
the myenteric plexus of the guinea-pig ileum. *J. Cell Biol.* 55:220a. (Abstr.)

Sano, K., Mayanagi, Y., Sekino, H., Ogashiwa, M., and Ishijima, B. (1970): Results   83
of stimulation and destruction of the posterior hypothalamus in man. *J.
Neurosurg.* 33:689-707.

Satoh, M. and Takagi, H. (1971a): Enhancement by morphine of the central   23
descending inhibitory influence on spinal sensory transmission. *Eur. J. Pharmacol.* 14:60-65.

Satoh, M. and Takagi, H. (1971b): Further observation on the enhancement by   23
morphine of the central descending inhibitory influence on spinal sensory
transmission. *Jap. J. Pharmacol.* 21:671-672.

Schild, H.O. (1957): Drug antagonism and pA_x. *Pharmacol. Rev.* 9:242-246.   65

Schulz, R., Cartwright, C., and Goldstein, A. (1974): Reversibility of morphine   110
tolerance and dependence in guinea-pig brain and myenteric plexus. *Nature*
251:329-331.

Schulz, R. and Goldstein, A. (1973): Morphine tolerance and supersensitivity to   109
5-hydroxytryptamine in the myenteric plexus of the guinea-pig. *Nature*
244:168-170.

Segal, D.S., Knapp, S., Kuczenski, R.T., and Mandell, A.J. (1973): The effects of
environmental isolation on behavior and regional rat brain tyrosine hydroxylase
and tryptophan hydroxylase activities. *Behav. Biol.* 8:47-53.

Shen, F.-H., Loh, H.H., and Way, E.L. (1970): Brain serotonin turnover in
morphine tolerant and dependent mice. *J. Pharmacol. Exp. Ther.* 175:427-434.

Simon, E.J. (1973): In search of the opiate receptor. *Am. J. Med. Sci.*
266:160-168.

Simon, E.J., Dole, W.P., and Hiller, J.M. (1972): Coupling of a new, active morphine derivative to sepharose for affinity chromatography. *Proc. Nat. Acad. Sci.* 69:1835-1837.

Simon, E.J., Hiller, J.M., and Edelman, I. (1973): Stereospecific binding of the   26,44,108
potent narcotic analgesic [^{3}H] etorphine to rat-brain homogenate. *Proc. Nat. Acad. Sci.* 70:1947-1949.

Simon, E.J., Hiller, J.M., Groth, J., and Edelman, I. (1975): Further properties of   45,46,47,
stereospecific opiate binding sites in rat brain: on the nature of the sodium   49
effect. *J. Pharmacol. Exp. Ther.* (In press)

Skultety, F.M. (1963): Stimulation of periaqueductal gray and hypothalamus.   91
Arch. Neurol. 8:608-620.

Snedecor, G.W. (1956): *Statistical Methods.* 5th Ed. Ames, Iowa: Iowa State   130
College Press.

Snyder, S.H., Young, A.B., Bennett, J.P., and Mulder, A.H. (1973): Synaptic
biochemistry of amino acids. *Fed. Proc.* 32:2039-2047.

Soto, E.F., Pasquini, J.M., Plácido, R., and La Torre, J.L. (1969): Fractionation of   50
lipids and proteolipids from cat grey and white matter by chromatography on an
organophilic dextran gel. *J. Chromatogr.* 41:400-409.

Sullivan, J.L., Segal, D.S., Kuczenski, R.T., and Mandell, A.J. (1972): Propranolol-
induced rapid activation of rat striatal tyrosine hydroxylase concomitant with
behavioral depression. *Biol. Psychiatry* 4:193-203.

Swain, H.H. and Seevers, M.H. (1974): Evaluation of new compounds for   71
morphine-like physical dependence in the rhesus monkey. *Bull. Problems Drug
Dependence* 36(Addendum):1168-1195.

Sweet, W.H. (1959): Pain. *In: Handbook of Physiology, Vol. 1, Sec. 1. Neuro-
physiology.* Magoun, H.W., ed. Baltimore: Williams and Wilkins, pp. 459-506.

Sweet, W.H. (1967): Neurosurgical management of pain. *In: New Concepts in Pain
and Its Clinical Management.* Way, E.L., ed. Philadelphia: F.A. Davis Co.,
pp. 169-185.

Swets, J.A. (1973): The relative operating characteristic in psychology. *Science*   81
182:990-1000.

Tagliamonte, A., Tagliamonte, P., Forn, J., Perez-Cruet, J., Krishna, G., and Gessa,   115
G.L. (1971): Stimulation of brain serotonin synthesis by dibutyryl-cyclic AMP
in rats. *J. Neurochem.* 18:1191-1196.

Takemori, A.E. (1973): Determination of pharmacological constants: Use of   66
narcotic antagonists to characterize analgesic receptors. *In: Advances in
Biochemical Psychopharmacology, Vol. 8. Narcotic Antagonists.* Braude, M.C.,
Harris, L.S., May, E.L., Smith, J.P., and Villarreal, J.E., eds. New York: Raven
Press, pp. 335-344.

164

Takemori, A.E., Oka, T., and Nishiyama, N. (1973): Alteration of analgesic receptor-antagonist interaction induced by morphine. *J. Pharmacol. Exp. Ther.* 186:261-265.   66,74

Terenius, L. (1972): Specific uptake of narcotic analgesics by subcellular fractions of the guinea-pig ileum. *Acta Pharmacol. Toxicol.* 31(Suppl.):50.   29,41

Terenius, L. (1973a): Characteristics of the "receptor" for narcotic analgesics in synaptic plasma membrane fraction from rat brain. *Acta Pharmacol. Toxicol.* 33:377-384.   26

Terenius, L. (1973b): Stereospecific interaction between narcotic analgesics and a synaptic plasma membrane fraction of rat cerebral cortex. *Acta Pharmacol. Toxicol.* 32:317-320.   26,39

Terenius, L. (1973c): Stereospecific uptake of narcotic analgesics by a subcellular fraction of the guinea-pig ileum. *Upsala J. Med. Sci.* 78:150-152.   29,40,41

Terenius, L. (1974a): Contribution of 'receptor' affinity to analgesic potency. *J. Pharm. Pharmacol.* 26:146-148.   40

Terenius, L. (1974b): A rapid assay of affinity for the narcotic receptor in rat brain: Application to methadone analogues. *Acta Pharmacol. Toxicol.* 34:88-91.   39,40,41

Terenius, L. and Wahlström, A. (1974): Inhibitor(s) of narcotic receptor binding in brain extracts and cerebrospinal fluid. *Acta Pharmacol. Toxicol.* 35(Suppl.):55. (Abstr.)   42

Teschemacher, Hj., Schubert, P., and Herz, A. (1973): Autoradiographic studies concerning the supraspinal site of the antinociceptive action of morphine when inhibiting the hindleg flexor reflex in rabbits. *Neuropharmacology* 12:123-131.

Tseng, L.F., Loh, H.H., Ho, I.K., and Way, E.L. (1974): The role of brain catecholamines in naloxone induced withdrawal in morphine dependent rats. *Proc. West. Pharmacol. Soc.* 17:178-183.   116

Tsou, K. and Jang, C.S. (1964): Studies on the site of analgesic action of morphine by intracerebral micro-injection. *Sci. Sinica* 13:1099-1109.   87

Tulunay, F.C. and Takemori, A.E. (1974a): Further studies on the alteration of analgesic receptor-antagonist interaction induced by morphine. *J. Pharmacol. Exp. Ther.* 190:401-407.   67

Tulunay, F.C. and Takemori, A.E. (1974b): The increased efficacy of narcotic antagonists induced by various narcotic analgesics. *J. Pharmacol. Exp. Ther.* 190:395-400.   67

Ungerstedt, U. (1971a): Histochemical studies on the effect of intracerebral and intraventricular injections of 6-hydroxydopamine on monoamine neurons in the rat brain. *In: 6-Hydroxydopamine and Catecholamine Neurons.* Malmfors, T. and Thoenen, H., eds. Amsterdam: North-Holland Publishing Co., pp. 101-127.   117

Ungerstedt, U. (1971b): Stereotaxic mapping of the monoamine pathways in the rat brain. *Acta Physiol. Scand.* Suppl. 367:1-48.   117

Vigouret, J., Teschemacher, Hj., Albus, K., and Herz, A. (1973): Differentiation between spinal and supraspinal sites of action of morphine when inhibiting the hindleg flexor reflex in rabbits. *Neuropharmacology* 12:111-121.

Villarreal, J.E. (1973): The effects of morphine agonists and antagonists on morphine-dependent rhesus monkeys. *In: Agonist and Antagonist Actions of Narcotic Analgesic Drugs.* Kosterlitz, H.W., Collier, H.O.J., and Villarreal, J.E., eds. Baltimore: University Park Press, pp. 73-93.

Villarreal, J.E. and Seevers, M.H. (1972): Evaluation of new compounds for morphine-like physical dependence in the rhesus monkey. *Bull. Problems Drug Dependence* 34(Addendum 7):1040-1053.   71

Watanabe, H. (1971): The development of tolerance to and of physical dependence on morphine following intraventricular injection in the rat. *Jap. J. Pharmacol.* 21:383-391.

Way, E.L. (1971): Cannabis prelude. *Pharmacol. Rev.* 23:263-264.

Way, E.L. (1972): Role of serotonin in morphine effects. *Fed. Proc.* 31:113-120.

Way, E.L. (1973): Brain neurohormones in morphine tolerance and dependence. *In: Pharmacology and the Future of Man, Vol. 1. Drug Abuse and Contraception.* (Proceedings of the 5th International Congress on Pharmacology, San Francisco, July 1972.) Cochin, J., ed. Basel: S. Karger, pp. 77-94.   112

Way, E.L. and Adler, T.K. (1962): The biological disposition of morphine and its surrogates. *Bull. Wld. Hlth. Org.* 26:51-66.   28

Way, E.L., Loh, H.H., and Shen, F.-H. (1969): Simultaneous quantitative assessment of morphine tolerance and physical dependence. *J. Pharmacol. Exp. Ther.* 167:1-8.   141

Way, E.L. and Shen, F.H. (1971): Catecholamines and 5-hydroxytryptamine. *In: Narcotic Drugs: Biochemical Pharmacology.* Clouet, D.H., ed. New York: Plenum Press, pp. 229-253.   95

Wei, E., Loh, H.H., and Way, E.L. (1972): Neuroanatomical correlates of morphine dependence. *Science* 177:616-617.

Wei, E., Loh, H.H., and Way, E.L. (1973a): Brain sites of precipitated abstinence in morphine-dependent rats. *J. Pharmacol. Exp. Ther.* 185:108-115.   92

Wei, E., Loh, H.H., and Way, E.L. (1973b): Quantitative aspects of precipitated abstinence in morphine-dependent rats. *J. Pharmacol. Exp. Ther.* 184:398-403.

Weiss, B. and Laties, V.G. (1970): The psychophysics of pain and analgesia in animals. *In: Animal Psychophysics: The Design and Conduct of Sensory Experiments.* Stebbins, W.C., ed. New York: Appleton-Century-Crofts, pp. 185-210.   88

Page

White, J.C. and Sweet, W.H. (1955): *Pain: Its Mechanisms and Neurosurgical Control.* Springfield, Ill.: C.C Thomas.

White, J.C. and Sweet, W.H. (1969): *Pain and the Neurosurgeon: A Forty-Year Experience.* Springfield, Ill.: C.C Thomas.   83

WHO Expert Committee on Addiction-Producing Drugs. Seventh Report (1957):   18
Wld. Hlth. Org. techn. Rep. Ser. 116:9.

WHO Expert Committee on Addiction-Producing Drugs. Thirteenth Report (1964):
Wld. Hlth. Org. techn. Rep. Ser. 273:9.

WHO Expert Committee on Drug Dependence. Sixteenth Report (1969): *Wld.*   19
Hlth. Org. techn. Rep. Ser. 407.

WHO Scientific Group on the Evaluation of Dependence-Producing Drugs (1964): 20
Wld. Hlth. Org. techn. Rep. Ser. 287.

Wikler, A., Norrell, H., and Miller, D. (1972): Limbic system and opioid addiction
in the rat. *Exp. Neurol.* 34:543-557.

Wilson, H.A., Pasternak, G.W., and Snyder, S.H. (1975a): Differentiation of opiate   138,139
agonist and antagonist receptor binding by protein modifying reagents. *Nature*
253:448-450.

Wilson, R.S., Rogers, M.E., Pert, C.B., and Snyder, S.H. (1975b): A homologous   28,29,62
series of analgesics: Correlation of receptor binding with analgesic potency. *J.*
Med. Chem. (In press)

Wolfle, T.L., Mayer, D.J., Carder, B., and Liebeskind, J.C. (1971): Motivational
effects of electrical stimulation in dorsal tegmentum of the rat. *Physiol. Behav.*
7:569-574.

Wong, D.T. and Horng, J.S. (1973): Stereospecific interaction of opiate narcotics in   27
binding of ³H-dihydromorphine to membranes of rat brain. *Life Sci.*
13:1543-1556.

Yamamura, H.I., Kuhar, M.J., Greenberg, D., and Snyder, S.H. (1974): Muscarinic
cholinergic receptor binding: regional distribution in monkey brain. *Brain Res.*
66:541-546.

Young, A.B. and Snyder, S.H. (1974a): The glycine synaptic receptor: evidence   140
that strychnine binding is associated with the ionic conductance mechanism.
Proc. Nat. Acad. Sci. 71:4002-4005.

Young, A.B. and Snyder, S.H. (1974b): Strychnine binding in rat spinal cord   140
membranes associated with the synaptic glycine receptor: cooperativity of
glycine interactions. *Mol. Pharmacol.* 10:790-809.

INDEX

iv